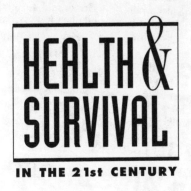

HEALTH & SURVIVAL

IN THE 21st CENTURY

*"The first step in philosophy is not a step;
The first step in philosophy is to open your eyes."*
W. Macneile Dixon
(*The Human Situation*, 1937)

THE COURIER MAIL 31.8.90

Hepatitis virus baffles doctors

SYDNEY.— ... blood do- ... ew strain ... which i ... nic live

United States National Institute of Health said doctors were confused over how it was transmitted.

... that drug addicts ... ndles but

THE COURIER MAIL 5.4.89

Cancer deaths up 14pc

DEATHS from cancer increased by 14.2 per cent between 1978 and ...

Health costs soar

WASHINGTON: The cost of health care in the US is rising quickly and soon Americans will pay mor... ... lion dollars ... tors ...

a tril- doc- ling ay. of

12.12.91

THE AUSTRALIAN 20.5.91

Disease more rampant now than 20 years ago

By science and technology writer JULIAN CRIBB

AUSTRALIANS are suffering from far more chronic diseases and infections than they did a decade ago ...

handicap, lion who a Australi bound to because tion and vices we cope wit illness, E "Austr not well ould s ay," he Envir ere th n thm

More die of bowel cancer

THE death rate from bowel cancer was increasing in Queensland, the State Health Minister, Mrs Harvey, said yesterday.

Bowel cancer ... second

THE COURIER MAIL 11.2.88

Elderly on drugs, an 'epidemic'

ABUSE of prescribed drugs by elderly Australians was a "hidden epidemic", a Drug-Arm spokesman said yesterday.

The Queensland manager, Mr Chris Levy, said many people over 60 were dependent on tranquillisers.

A recent ...vey by the Australian Consumer Association showed tranquillisers were prescribed for an average period of six years, even though the recommended period was about three weeks.

One person had been taking prescribed tranquillisers for 22 years.

The survey revealed respondents over 60 were taking on average five different prescribed drugs at any one time.

THE COURIER MAIL 3.4.89

Melanoma out of control: expert

By MARGARET HARRIS
Medical Writer

The rate of melanoma amo... Australians has doubled in ... past 10 years and the death rat... continuing to rise, according t... leading Melbourne dermatolog... ...can... ...uld be prudent ...r people to reduce their ...take of fat and increase ...fibre in their diets," she said.

16.5.91 THE HERALD MORNING

THE COURIER MAIL 9.8.90

Brain disease on way to epidemic: expert

AUSTRALIAN adults had a one in eight chance of Alzheimer's disease or a related disorder, an expert said yesterday.

Alzheimer's Association president Dr Henry Brodaty said the number of victims was increasing faster than in Canada New Zealand

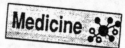

Medicine

Dr Brodaty said Australia's present level of research funding represented "about 8¢ per

cover the structure of abnormal protein in the brains of Alzheimer' sufferers, he said.

"We urgently need to understand the causes of Alzheimer's disease, how to prevent it, how to treat d how best to care for sufferers and their ies."

THE AUSTRALIAN 6.7.91

Killer diseases re-emerge

INFECTIOUS diseases long regarded as of little threat ere re-emerging around the orld, a visiting United States esearcher said yesterday.

Dr Frederick Murphy, of the entres for Disease Control n Atlanta, said cholera and engue fever were spreading.

Cholera epidemics had reently swept Latin Ame

Dengue fever was a the rise and had been ted in northern Austra

Diseases could rema stant or be "eradicate "something can hap trigger a new epidem as a change in an org human behaviour.

AIDS was still the

THE AUSTRALIAN 16.6.91

Painkiller buying habit tops $100 million a year

AUSTRALIANS spend ore than $100 million a year n over-the-counter painki rs, most of which are pu hased from supermarket ccording to the Australi onsumers' Association.

Consumers frequently p: high prices for brand nan and market leaders, wl per analgesics conta ical ingredie ice ma

The report found one supermarket brand of para-

THE AUSTRALIAN 11.5.91

Children 'using more painkillers'

SCHOOL children are drinking and smoking less but using more painkillers, according to a report released in Adelaide yesterday.

The report — Survey of Alcohol, Tobacco and other Drug Use by South Australian School Child

THE COURIER MAIL 13·11·91

Malaria on the rise

SYDNEY: Malaria is on the increase in Australia and authorities have been warned to remain vigilant to prevent the disease from re-establishing itself.

The Australian Malaria 012 cases were

ly Papua New Guinea.

Dr Hall said Australia was declared malaria-free in 1981 but the mosquitoes that spread the disease were still active in the north.

"The first point is that we want to ensure that it doesn't get re-established here," he

THE AUSTRALIAN 19.8.91
d to maintain

Cancer leading killer of men

SALLY HOPMAN

NCER has replaced heart se as the main killer of alian men, being reble for almost 27 per male deaths.

e 64,660 male deaths red in 1990, 17,300 were related, according to released by the Aust Bureau of Sta

However heart disease remained the biggest killer responsible for 25.2 per cent of all female deaths.

The latest bureau figures showing cancer as the main killer took the executive director of the Cancer C Elain

Ms Henry said people wer often frightened when hit by "shock" statistics.

"They take the wrong attitude by thinking it is inevita ble they will get

Hospital chief dies of heart attack at 54

THE COURIER 22.10.91

By JO

ONE of Q
ing paedit
Father of th
a heart atta
field home

The med
ent of the
Hospital, D
54, died on
launch of o
ects, the
station. Ra

Dr Fras
Brisbane a
the Ang
Grammar

He grad
University
the early
studied in
returned

Arthritis medication 'life-threatening'

THE AUSTRALIAN 27.8.90

THE majority of Australians suffering arthritis are being wrongly prescribed long-term medication which could result in life-threatening complications from stomach ulcers.

A significant number of arthritis sufferers taking non-steroidal anti-inflammatory drugs (NSAIDs) over a 30-year period will suffer

could bring on life-threatening complications without warning.

He said United States studies had shown that 60 per cent of those who developed potentially fatal complications arising from an NSAID-induced ulcer had no advance warning like pain or bleedin

four pa
ulcers
NSAIDs
utiating
warning
ms.

Brooks,
North
NSAIDs
ed

Estrogen linked to breast cancer risk

THE COURIER MAIL 20.4.91

WASHINGTON: Menopausal women who take the hormone estrogen for 15 years or more face a 30 percent higher risk of breast cancer, the Centre for Disease Control says.

But women who use the drug for five years or less apparently have no increased risk at all.

The CDC findings, re
in the Journal of t
Medical
bas

a family history of breast cancer who use estrogen for any amount of time face a risk more than 200 percent greater.

For women who bega
the hormone
premenon
inc

Wave of tuberculosis swamps New Yorkers

THE COURIER MAIL 13.7.91

NEW YORK: Tuberculosis, a disease thought to have been largely eradicated in the stern world since the is swamping New

case but in at least three cases it has spread to general wards.

The spread comes as a grap example of the way in which First and Third worlds live by-side in the teeming str New York.

Health authorities ha
the outbreak to three f
new influx of Third
ants, particularly fro
aiti; the expanding
many of them
addicted to
d the

previous year.
e expect-
ses

homeless has stret
health budget to bre

The bacterial inf
no longer fata
d with mod

the p
tals is
se to u
the st
d thei
their

So fa
ave be
solate
signe
sion

Children get fat

WASHINGTON: America's children were fatter, more suicidal, more murderous and scored lower on standardised tests in th past few years than in the 1960s, researchers reported yesterday.

The Courier Mail 4.1.92

Now t
to build new
New York alrea
avest budget crisis s
70s and among the p
rocketing cost of
concer

THE AUSTRALIAN 19.8.91

Third of children at risk from high cholesterol

MORE than a third of Australian children could be at high risk of future heart and artery disease because they have too much cholesterol in their blood, according to the findings of a study.

Cholesterol screening of 1112 school children, aged between 10 and 12, revealed that more than 50 per cent of children tested had levels above that recommended by the National Heart Foundation.

Up to 36 per cent of boys and 39 per cent of girls were identified as being at risk with high levels of cholesterol.

About 2̶̶̶̶

Foundation is 4.5 millimolles per litre of blood.

One girl in the test registered a level of 8.1̶ units per litre.

"The distribution of cholesterol levels in Australian children compares unfavourably with distributions in children in countries with low rates of cardiovascular disease and indicates a need for widespread, appropriate diet and lifestyle changes," the study concludes.

World Health Organisation experts say an ̶̶̶̶l level would be 3.1 units.

disquieting data parallel̶ ̶ecent data on Australian̶ during the 1989 National̶ ̶ion risk factor prevalence̶ ̶r Vandongen said.

7 per cent of men and 39̶ ̶men were found to have̶ ̶rol levels of 5.5 or more –̶ ̶l as being higher then̶

THE COURIER MAIL 20.2.91

Hospital gets Big Macs

MELBOURNE: The McDonald's fast food chain wants to follow an American trend and sell its hamburgers in hospitals.

This follows a decision by Melbourne's Royal Children's Hospital to allow the chain to open a $1 million restaurant in soon-to-be-completed extensions.

"Where people congregate, people eat — why shouldn't we be there?" ̶̶̶̶̶ald's vice-president yesterday̶

At least 12 United States hospitals have McDonald's restaurants.

Although no firm plans have been ̶̶̶̶̶̶̶ said: "We are ̶̶̶̶̶̶ pita̶ foo̶ vie̶ ha̶ w̶

su̶ n̶

Increase in number of diabetics

̶̶̶̶̶portion of Austra-̶̶̶̶̶̶̶bed

The C̶̶̶̶̶ THE SYDNEY ̶̶̶̶ 13.9.90

Melanoma is 'out of control', doctor says

By MARGARET HARRIS
Medical Reporter

Melanoma, a major killer of young Australian women, is increasing at such a rapid rate, dermatologists now believe it may be caused by more than simply sun exposure.

Dr Alan Cooper, the honorary secretary of the Australasian College of Dermatologists, said many more people were developing the lethal skin tumour than researchers expected. "It is out of control," he said. "The rate of increase is really frightening."

By 1985 the number of cases had reached levels dermatol̶̶̶̶ thought they w̶̶̶̶̶̶ said̶̶̶

the symposium that the incidence of melanomas in NSW had probably doubled over the past 10 years, but that sunlight was probably to blame for less than half the cases.

Other papers presented to the symposium have revealed that US researchers have been forced to drastically increase their earlier predictions of the future incidence of melanomas.

Dr Cooper said melanoma̶ the sixth most ̶̶̶̶̶̶ Alt̶̶̶̶̶̶

s.

̶t of
̶7-78,

̶meta-
̶d and
̶uction

̶re like-

By the same author
Beat Heart Disease
Let's Live A Lot
The Grasshopper Aircraft Operating Manual
Health Facts Prove The Pritikin Program
The Health Revolution
The New Health Revolution
The Health Revolution Cookbook
The Health Revolution, Third Edition
The Anti-Heart Attack, Anti-Cancer Cookbook
The Health Revolution, Fourth Edition
Improving on Pritikin

HEALTH & SURVIVAL

IN THE 21st CENTURY

⚘ROSS HORNE

MARGARET
Gee

Published by
Margaret Gee Publishing
an imprint of
Margaret Gee Holdings
Suite 2a, 61 Victoria Street, McMahons Point, 2060
A.C.N. 005 604 464

First published in 1992

Distributed by Gary Allen Pty Ltd
9 Cooper Street, Smithfield, NSW, 2164

National Library of Australia
Cataloguing-in-Publication entry

Horne, Ross
    Health & survival in the 21st century.
    Bibliography.
    ISBN 1 875574 07 7.

    1. Medicine, Preventive. 2. Self-care, Health. I. Title.
613

Typeset by Midland Typesetters, Victoria
Printed by Australian Print Group, Victoria

To Joan and Mike

Contents

Acknowledgments

This book is a compilation of a great many facts assembled together like pieces of a jigsaw puzzle in an attempt to form a complete picture.

Although facts are unalterable, they can be interpreted in different ways, and often an incorrect interpretation, unchallenged, becomes mistakenly accepted as the truth. And when such a false fact is mixed among the real facts as pieces of the jigsaw (sometimes getting stretched a bit to make it fit), confusion is inevitable, leading to further mistakes. Realizing this, two approaches to the puzzle must therefore be adopted; first, the false pieces must be identified and discarded, and then the remaining true pieces must be fitted together.

This is what I have tried to do, acting as it were as chairman of a brainstorming session, the members of which are the people whose names appear in the chapters that follow. Each of these thinking individuals, past and present, have contributed to clarify the emerging picture, the genuineness of which is displayed by the harmony with which the separate pieces fit together.

Not many of these outstanding people have received the recognition due to them, and in most cases their achievements, considered "oddball" by the rank and file, have been ignored. Such is the lot of everybody who comes up with unusual ideas, and this is fair enough, because in human affairs, oddballs are potentially more dangerous than plodders, while their unusual ideas, if really sound, eventually win through. Whether my characters deserve the credit I pay them, readers can decide for themselves.

Even greater credit is due to researchers forced to go

it alone when rejected by lesser mortals and repressed by ignorant "powers that be". Names like Bechamp, Kuhne, De Lacy Evans, Densmore, Bell, Dewey, Tilden, Gerson, Koch, Moerman, Howell, Shelton, Hoxsey, Rabinowitch, Morrison, Pritikin and Mendelsohn come to mind from out of the past.

But it is the present-day champions of the truth who most urgently need our acknowledgment and support as they strive to free the medical profession from its straitjacket of dogma and ignorance. Gradually they are succeeding. In the field of heart disease the medical professionals are now adopting the ideas of Nathan Pritikin they not long ago ridiculed, and in the field of cancer they are beginning to tune in to Max Gerson's methods for natural remissions of cancer, still successfully being demonstrated by Dr Gerson's daughter, Charlotte, of the Gerson Institute in California.

Fighting hardest against "the forces of agnosticism" (as Professor Otto Warburg called them) in the field of AIDS are people like Professor Peter Duesberg, Professor Robert Roote-Bernstein, Dr Joan McKenna, Dr Laurence Badgley, Dr Joe Sonnerbend, Dr Michael Culbert, and journalists John Lauritsen and Jad Adams. To these steadfast individuals I wish to give special acknowledgment for the information they have provided me and for their kind permission to quote them liberally. These people are made of the "right stuff" and in my estimation rate with the fighter pilots of the Battle of Britain in that when *their* fight is over it will be said of them: "Never before in the field of human conflict has so much been owed by so many to so few."

Author's Preface

When a man's science exceedeth his sense,
He perishes by his ignorance.

Oriental Proverb

Viewed from space today, **Planet Earth** looks little different from how it would have looked a thousand years ago. Oceans and continents clearly visible in technicolor, veiled in swirling wisps of white clouds—it makes a pretty picture.

Closer inspection, however, reveals big changes: less forest land, more deserts, more smoke haze, more scars. Damage, man-made.

But that's only the visible damage. There is far more damage that you cannot see: the Earth's remaining soil is depleted in life-sustaining minerals, the oceans are polluted and depleted in marine life, and many species of animals and trees have vanished.

Humans have been gradually destroying our planet for thousands of years, but with the discovery of oil and the internal combustion engine, accompanied with the human population explosion, the destruction over the last hundred years has brought about a situation nearing total disaster. And still the numbers increase, still the "national economies" expand, still we exhort greater efforts for "productivity". It's as if we are all passengers on a speeding *Titanic*, equipped with modern radar that the captain doesn't understand. The warning is there, loud and clear, but the crew is pre-occupied with attending to the comfort of the passengers.

"Those whom the gods wish to destroy, they first

make mad"—Euripides (485–406 BC) has been quoted many times since uttering those words. Bertrand Russell (1872–1970) put it a different way when he made the prediction that "man's half-cleverness would be the means of his own destruction . . ."

Are we mad? Or just "half-clever"? It doesn't matter: the final result will be the same, and already the future of the next few generations is a most uncertain one, even for those in the most favored circumstances.

The 21st Century will undoubtedly witness the resolution of the world's overpopulation problem, and because the problem is, despite our best efforts to solve it, getting worse instead of better, it is inevitable that the matter will be resolved in the same manner by which other kinds of plagues have been terminated in the past.

Food is the main limiting factor, not only the quantity of it but also the quality—a fact that is making itself felt today where more people in the world die of semi-starvation on a full stomach than those that die of complete starvation on an empty stomach. (By semi-starvation I mean malnutrition-related diseases due to poor quality food, a topic which forms the main theme of this book.)

In the more distant past when major upheavals of various kinds have upset the equilibrium of the Earth's various inhabitants, some species have become extinct while others, purged of their weak, have improved. Out of this rigorous process emerged the human race, which has survived and flourished by virtue not of physical strength but of mental strength. It is the fittest that survive, and in human affairs fitness for survival is measured in terms of mental capacity.

It is a mistake to measure mental capacity simply on a person's degree of success in financial or academic circles; a more reliable indicator is the state of their physical health and their general philosophy on life. It does not display great intelligence to make a fortune only to be worried about your health and maybe die of a heart attack or some other avoidable disease.

Most "diseases of civilization" are avoidable, and the

Western world's vast and increasing health problems today are a reflection of the ignorance and "half-cleverness" of our supposedly well-informed leaders and medical technocrats, together with the money-making aspirations of the food manufacturers and the pharmaceutical industry.

Thus, while it is all very well to feel compassion for diseased and starving populations elsewhere in the world, and to condescendingly send them food supplies so they can continue to live and breed, it should not be assumed that we are a great deal better off ourselves. To repeat: food is the major factor in health and survival, and the widespread health problems we have are direct reflections of the biochemical quality of our food. As our soil becomes more and more depleted, as our food becomes more and more manufactured, so our bodies display the evidence. Death by heart attack, cancer, asthma or diabetes is as final as that from starvation.

Our immediate problems at home stemming from poor nutrition in the midst of plenty we must deal with if we are to survive as a healthy nation. Our medical experts are failing to deal with these problems because they don't understand them, so we must get to understand and deal with them ourselves. Self-preservation is an instinct that overrides all others—self-preservation and the preservation of our offspring. It is an instinct that works best with open

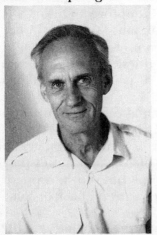

eyes and an alert mind. Whatever the adversity faced with now or in the future, we can best survive if we know what to expect and how to deal with it.

Some of the information that follows may surprise you—in fact, I bet it will—but it will help you survive.

Happy landings,
Ross Horne

Foreword

by Professor John Wright

About twenty years ago, Ross Horne, then a senior captain and instructor on jumbo jets with Qantas Airways, introduced to Australia the ideas of Nathan Pritikin, a retired electronics engineer from California. The ideas concerned diet and its relationship with the various health problems of modern society, a subject about which, over those twenty years, Mr Horne has extended his concept, seeking always to find a unifying theme for maintaining good health.

The medical profession has a long history of discomfort with health recommendations coming from non-professionals. It would be a great pity if Ross Horne's quest for truth and his abiding concern for his fellow man should draw a response of intolerance or condescension from conventional medicine, particularly in view of the fact that conventional medicine has arrived at an impasse that may indicate the present system is not achieving the desired results.

Health costs rocket up at rates exceeding population growth by a factor of fifteen times. Ever-more refined equipment finds exactly the same diseases but at greater cost. Conventional medical management largely fails in controlling, treating or achieving improvement in many areas of illness.

This book is devoted to the subject of total health care in the belief that all illness is avoidable and should never be tolerated in themselves by intelligent people. In this book, Mr Horne has reviewed and demonstrated the beliefs of many very distinguished medical scientists and doctors, past and present, and has attempted to perceive patterns that are not readily apparent to those of conventional medical upbringing. Above that, he has the ability to anticipate the questions and doubts which trouble the whole population, and he has the knack of presenting solutions with an appealing simplicity.

As in his previous writings, Ross Horne demonstrates here his remarkable scholarship and diligence, coherence and worldly wisdom. Insofar as his message may contain truths which have escaped conventional teaching, particularly in the area of nutrition and its influence on body systems and pathology, then he has demonstrated a serious deficiency in awareness that exists in so-called well-informed circles.

Many would view this sort of book as required reading for medical students, not only because they must learn to very carefully analyse, agree with or refute the claims he makes, but also because medical students should graduate knowing what sorts of questions their patients will increasingly ask them and why so many of the sick and troubled will increasingly depart from adherence to conventional practitioners.

Medical students of the future may also find it remarkable that the unifying principles brought together in this book have been preached by distinguished medical scholars for hundreds of years. The wonder is that the maturation of these ideas has not yet led to a realistic review of the immense sociologic and civilisational aspects of health delivery. Ultimately, it seems a matter of social, political and medical morality.

I have read this book with the same sense of embarrassment as will most of my medical colleagues—that I have not known answers to so many of the questions which he asks, nearly forty-five years after I began as a medical student. Above all, I am fearful and saddened that, if too many of my colleagues are intolerant of the great themes about which Ross Horne writes, refusing to give them long second thoughts, then in another forty-five years other doctors will still be fearful and saddened, and countless millions of humans may have been deprived of their birthright.

This is a very disturbing book. Ross Horne is asking us all to at least hear the beat of a different drum. The peoples and patients of this world are asking the same question.

The crescendo anthem is lucid, simple, stimulating and unmistakably hopeful. Our medical ancestors, through this book, call us to listen again and again.

John Wright
MB BS FRACS FACS
Surgeon, Professorial Staff U.N.S.W. 1963–87;
now Consultant Surgeon, Sydney.

Foreword

to *The Health Revolution*
by Dr Dean Burk

(A foundation member of the US National Cancer Institute and former head of the Institute's Cytochemistry Department, Dr Burk is best known for his work on cancer research for which he has received honors from France, Britain, Germany and Russia. Formerly Associate Professor of Biochemistry, Cornell University, he has worked in cancer research at the Kaiser Wilhelm Institute in Germany and at the Russian Academy of Science, Moscow. Dr Burk is the recipient of the Domagk Prize for cancer research, a Knight Commander of the medical Order of Bethlehem, and a Knight of the Mark Twain Society. He is co-author of the books Cancer, Approaches to Tumor Chemotherapy *and* Cell Chemistry, *and author of over 250 published scientific papers.)*

Having spent most of my professional life in the field of cancer research—a field of great complexity and no little confusion—I was astonished and delighted to become acquainted with this book.

My astonishment arises from the discovery that a layman (the author is a retired airline captain) should have gained such a comprehensive understanding of the complex biological processes which lead to the disease called cancer and to be able to describe these processes in a manner easily understandable by other laymen.

The author describes the origins of not only cancer but of other so-called diseases of civilization and the natural measures required to avoid and control them.

When it is considered that few medical professionals possess this knowledge, this is no mean achievement.

The strength, integrity and happiness of a nation are directly proportional to the state of health of its citizens. In the distant past civilizations have risen, flourished and declined, their ruins covered by desert sands. Did affluence destroy them? Are we heading the same way?

Perhaps humans are too clever for their own good. In the pursuit of progress and pleasure they at the same time sow the seeds of their own destruction.

Modern man must comprehend the message presented in this book that the greatest threat to his survival is not that of nuclear war, because although that threat is real, at least everyone is aware of it. The threat most dangerous to mankind comes from the destroyers active right now, subtle and unseen—the poisoning of our soil and water supplies, the de-naturing of our food, the ever-increasing destruction of the environment.

No more do people die of old age; instead, heart attacks, strokes, cancer, diabetes and so on are today accepted as normal causes of death. Influenza, arthritis, indigestion, constipation, aches and pains and medicine are a normal part of life. Are coronary bypasses, hysterectomies, reading glasses, hearing aids, wheelchairs, false teeth and plastic hip joints to be considered normal too?

On his long evolutionary journey, man has strayed on to dangerous ground. Now we are at a crossroads, and whichever way we take there will be some rough going. As ever, the fittest will survive.

Ross Horne's book is a survival manual for the trip ahead.

Dean Burk
Washington DC

Introduction

The history of mankind is an immense sea of errors in which a few obscure truths may here and there be found.

Cesare Beccaria

And don't kid yourself the 21st Century will be any different.

The author

The 21st Century lies ahead of us, and in it a lot of interesting things are going to happen, some of which you don't have to be a genius to foretell.

The course of human history has been one of fluctuating fortunes punctuated by triumphs and tragedies, successes and mistakes. For every triumph there would be at a guess a hundred tragedies, for every success, a hundred mistakes. From time to time a good idea backfires, and from time to time an established principle turns out to be a mistake. And that's how it goes: only by making mistakes and repairing them can progress be achieved.

Or at least what we have considered to be progress is achieved, but now we are having doubts because suddenly we have become aware we may have gone too far. We have "progressed" to a point where we have upset the equilibrium of our planet Earth, thereby threatening the survival of all its inhabitants.

"Those who do not learn by the mistakes of the past are condemned to repeat them" is an old proverb, and the fact that "history repeats itself" demonstrates that most of the time the mistakes of the past receive only temporary notice and are repeated over and over. Nothing is different today and many of today's crop of mistakes are common knowledge, more of a nuisance than a danger. But what is not common knowledge, not even in the ranks of our "better informed" citizens, is that, woven into our traditional day to day lifestyle, there are dangerous errors that are responsible for most of the current health problems in the world and for their ever-increasing severity. These errors, which are gradually becoming more evident, are the result of human over-confidence and gross ignorance of the fundamental laws of Nature. The ignorance has persisted so long because, obsessed with our fancied superiority of science and technology, we tend to disregard the simple as being beneath notice.

The world, sociologically, is divided into two groups: the haves and the have-nots. A great proportion of the have-nots live on or below the subsistence level and are perishing from disease and starvation, while to help them out a bit, the haves send them relief supplies of wheat and powdered milk.

This scenario is one of tremendous irony, because the affluent (have) nations who out of pity donate fourth-rate relief food to the suffering have-nots are, without realizing it, themselves suffering from malnutrition, of a different kind that is not obvious but which kills them off just as effectively, although not as quickly, as undernourishment kills off the poor.

When malnutrition is thought about, the picture that comes to mind is that of an emaciated child with hand outstretched and imploring eyes, a child destined for a life of disease if not death by starvation. It is a sad thought, but just as sad is it to observe our own "well-fed" children and to predict what the future holds for them. On present-day statistics, one in every three people will get cancer, one in every two will die of a circulatory disease, and the rest, if not killed in accidents, will perish from some other disease. The death certificates will show cause of death to be any of the above, but the real cause, if properly recorded, would read "degeneration caused by malnutrition", because it is defective nutrition supplied us by our traditional Western diet that underlies each and every one of the so-called diseases of civilization, not ignoring that smoking and alcohol play their part as well.

The human lifespan potential as agreed by contemporary scientists is 120 years. That this was known and recorded in ancient times is evidenced in the bible, Genesis VI.3: "And the Lord said, My spirit will not always strive with man, for that he also is flesh; yet his days shall be a hundred and twenty years." With an average life expectancy in modern society of only about seventy-five years, it's surprising that more people are not complaining about being short-changed. The explanation for this appears to be that our culture, which in the past was moulded on religious beliefs, has accepted the biblical lifespan of "three score years and ten", which reduced term was decreed by God consequentially to the sinful habits acquired by mankind. Seventy years or thereabouts is therefore more or less mistakenly taken as an acceptable life span.

Following from all this, it must be a reasonable assumption whether of either a religious or a scientific persuasion that if the errors in lifestyle with which we prematurely degenerate our bodies and minds are corrected, then a vast improvement to our individual life potential will follow.

That a situation could ever exist where all people live completely disease free with never a tooth cavity or even a pimple to spoil a happy lifetime is of course just a Utopian dream, because our bad habits are too deeply ingrained in our culture along with the transient pleasures that they bring, and along with the wishful but grossly mistaken thinking that modern medicine can conquer disease. Be that as it may, the behavior of the herd need be no concern of yours because it is also a fundamental rule of Nature that when things get desperate it's every man for himself, and the devil take the hindmost.

The things *are* desperate, the writing is on the wall.

As the news headlines proclaim daily, our health problems continue to increase. Old diseases once thought abolished are re-appearing, and rare ones are becoming common, all of them incurable by medical drugs. Cancer, asthma and arthritis are on the increase, and cardiovascular disease (heart/stroke) is still the major cause of death. Cancer, for which there is no effective medical treatment, is now responsible for one in four of all deaths and at the present rate of increase will soon account for one in three. And doctors can do nothing about it, dying as predictably as everybody else as the increasing cost of medicine threatens to bankrupt our economy.

That is how we stand at the threshold of the 21st Century. However, the chances of your personal survival and the survival of your children need not be assessed from this glum outlook, because with the right knowledge and the right application you can if you so wish raise your chances of a longer than average life span to record heights. Unfortunately, the right knowledge has not yet been discovered by our so-called experts on nutrition, who still propound the old concept of "the five basic food groups"*, which concept, invented many years ago by the US Department of Agriculture, does more good for the food industry and the medical industry than it does for the food consumers. The object of this book is to provide information on the subject that is up to date and to expose a lot of the false concepts pertaining not only to nutrition but to other aspects of our culture which greatly affect our health, not the least of which is the ever-increasing danger presented by pharmaceutical drugs and the people who dispense them.

Remember, whatever you do, that despite the wonderful advances in surgery and other crisis-dealing medicines, modern medical personnel have only a vague and usually erroneous understanding of the metabolic upsets that fill the Pandora's box of human diseases, and can therefore do little to help the chronically sick. Perhaps

* In the U.S.A. they classify the various foods into only four groups.

this statement from the famous English cancer specialist, Dr Kasper Blond, explains why:

"The problem must be considered as an insoluble medical problem because it is essentially a nutritional and social problem, in other words, a problem of prevention. Such a problem cannot be solved by animal experiments, vaccines and drugs. Statisticians, pathologists, biochemists and doctors cannot solve social problems."

To sum up this introduction and its emphasis on mistakes, the words of the famous Swedish doctor, Are Waerland, put it all in a nutshell: "We are not concerned with diseases but with mistakes . . . of living. Get rid of the mistakes and the diseases will disappear of their own accord."

CHAPTER 1

Health—
Your Birthright

There is no cure for birth or death save to enjoy the interval.

George Santayana

Health is the birthright of all living things in their natural environment. It is guaranteed by the laws of Nature while ever those laws are respected.

But we conceited humans, because we have dammed a few rivers and cut a few canals, have succeeded in deluding ourselves that we have mastered Nature. And because we have changed a few species of plants and animals to our advantage, and have invented heart transplants and so on, we further delude ourselves that we know better than Nature and can do better on our own. And that's why we have been deprived of our most precious birthright—good health from birth to old age.

In nature there are neither rewards or punishments. There are consequences.

Robert Ingersoll

It's as simple as that. People who are never sick and who live long are not lucky—they, knowingly or unknowingly, have merely followed habits of life in accord with Nature's simple guidelines. Their good health is not a reward, it is a consequence—natural and predictable. By the same token, people who get sick from time to time or even all of the time are not unlucky; they are not in any sense unfortunate victims of disease—their ill-health is merely a predictable consequence of things they are doing wrong.

The concept of natural health is simple and unshakeable, and can be proven in a very short space of time. The concept is:

1 Good health is the normal state of all living things and will always be maintained in the absence of unnatural influences.

2 In sound health, the defensive systems of the body are capable of easily repelling and destroying any potentially harmful organism (germ or virus) that may be encountered.

3 Disease of any kind (infectious or metabolic) can only eventuate if a person is subjected to adverse influences such as malnutrition, stress, etc, to the extent of exceeding the body's capacity to cope.

4 Providing the vital organs retain some function, then whatever the state of illness or injury, once the body is freed of the adverse influences responsible, it will immediately, without any outside help, commence to restore itself. And if at the same time optimum conditions of nutrition, sunshine, fresh air and rest are provided, the restoration will proceed at a surprisingly rapid rate.

These principles are fixed and unfailing, and can be observed working in any unspoiled environment in which trees, plants and animals exhibit constant vigorous health, and death occurs only through injury or old age.

Why do humans get sick? Why do we need doctors, dentists and hospitals? The human body in proper condition is as tough and germ resistant as that of any animal in the wild, and the only reason it becomes frail and susceptible to disease is that, in our civilized enclosures, we subject ourselves all the time to so many unnatural and harmful influences, the most harmful of them being the cooked and otherwise denaturalized food we eat. So with digestion overworked and with body chemistry not right, our health diminishes and symptoms of various malfunctions appear, such as head colds and blemishes in our early years, proceeding to the conventional problems of the middle aged and elderly.

Reclaiming Your Birthright

The key to reclaiming your birthright and powering your way back to topline health and vigor is not that you have to do anything very special. You don't need to buy lots of herbs or meditate or have acupuncture.

All you have to do is to STOP doing the things that are doing you harm, whereupon your body, given favorable circumstances and with its inbuilt wisdom, will soon restore itself.

That is simple—but there are pitfalls, the main one being that the world is full of conflicting advice, most of it either only half right and a lot of it totally wrong, which means you must sift all the information you are offered regardless of its source. Remember: opinions only become facts when they are proven. To demonstrate this point, the chapters which follow describe just how mistaken many of our traditional beliefs are—beliefs about nutrition, germs and viruses, disease and medicine—which misconceptions, while held on to, prevent any chance of a full comprehension of our subject. Other information follows as well, of course, and as Sherlock Holmes said to his friend Dr Watson (or words to the same effect): "When you have eliminated all that is false then whatever remains must be the truth."

CHAPTER 2

The *Milieu Interieur* (The Environment Within)

Bernard was right, the germ is nothing—the milieu is everything.

Louis Pasteur

There is great concern these days about the environment. We are at last realizing that human activity—farming, fishing, mining, manufacturing, etc—has steadily upset the balance of Nature and has already caused irreparable change to our world and the destruction of many forms of life. With forests destroyed, soil degraded, rivers, oceans and atmosphere polluted, Planet Earth is diseased and humans are the cause of it all.

The damage man has caused to the environment was not done maliciously, but out of ignorance, and the same applies to the damage man has caused—and still is causing—to himself with his personally destructive habits of living. This self-inflicted damage, more often than not put down to bad luck, is reflected in daily newspaper reports concerning the increasing problems of public health. The problem of declining public health is a problem of equal importance for humanity to the environmental issue, and the sooner people realize that they are themselves as much responsible for the welfare of their own bodies as they are for the welfare of the environment, the sooner both problems can be resolved.

When considering the health of the body as a whole, including the mind, it must first be understood that the body is made up of many billions of living cells, each one a separate, tiny, living organism which needs to be individually sustained. If each individual cell receives the nutrition and oxygen it needs and has its personal waste products removed, it will be healthy. And if every cell in the body is likewise healthy, then it follows that the entire body will be healthy too.

Thus total health can only be achieved by first attending to inner health, because the two are indivisible: they are one and the same.

To achieve a state in which the various organs of the body function as they are meant to, and are protected by a fully functional immune system, the environment within the body must be just right. The principle of total body health being directly related to the purity of the fluid environment in which the body cells dwell was conceived by the great 19th-Century physiologist Claude Bernard of France. Bernard coined the term *"milieu interieur"*, which in French means "environment within".

This gently flowing fluid is called extra-cellular fluid, or lymph, and consists of plasma, the clear liquid component of the blood, which seeps from the capillary vessels of the main blood circulation into the body tissues to deliver oxygen and nutrients to them and to convey the cells' waste products away for elimination. The "spent" lymph returns to the main blood circulation via a network of vessels similar to veins called the lymphatic system, propelled by the squeezing action that occurs with muscle movements of ordinary activity and better still by exercise of a more vigorous nature. The chemical composition of lymph is almost the same as seawater, which reflects the fact the cells of our bodies are descendants of the primitive single-celled animals of the sea which preceded the higher forms of life billions of years ago.

The purity of the *milieu interieur* therefore depends

on the quality of the blood and lymph and the vigor of the circulation, the cleansing action of the lymph being as important as its nourishing action. And, in turn, the quality of the blood is dependent primarily on the efficiency of the liver and kidneys and the quality of the food and water from which the body makes new blood.

When the quality of the *milieu interieur* is just right the blood and lymph flow freely, rich in nutrients and oxygen and free of unwanted substances or toxins; the red cells float freely and so too do the white cells of the immune system, vigorous and efficient. When this ideal condition is achieved, all the organs of the body harmonize and everything works the way it should. The condition of perfectly balanced body chemistry is called "homeostasis", a term coined by the great physiologist Walter Cannon, MD Sc.D, of Harvard University. In his famous book, *The Wisdom of the Body* (1932, W.W. Norton Publishers), Dr Cannon explained how, regardless of conditions that may vary widely, the "body wisdom" works constantly to maintain homeostasis.

If there are any deficiencies in nutrition, if there exists any form of pollution, or if there is inadequate oxygen or poor circulation or organ malfunction, the *milieu interieur* will suffer, and with it the health of the body. The nature of the milieu's degradation will affect the extent of upset to homeostasis and how the body will react. One way or another, the body will be ill at ease or "dis-eased", and according to whatever symptoms the body displays, so one or another of a textbook full of medical names will be given to it.

The most common and most serious form of degradation of the *milieu interieur* is toxemia caused by improper diet. In most cases the diet is reasonably adequate in necessary nutrients, but the problem of malnutrition nevertheless exists because of excesses of some components, the de-naturing effect of cooking and the inclusion of harmful substances such as salt, condiments and refined sugar, etc.

As toxemia can occur in countless different forms and

degrees, not only through improper diet but through stress, lack of fresh air and sunshine, etc, once the limits of "body wisdom" are exceeded the resultant effects may vary widely, which explains why there are so many different diseases listed in the medical textbooks and why doctors, not realizing the true nature of the problem, sometimes have so much difficulty deciding which disease is "attacking" their patient and which drug to "fight" it with.

When the usual blood tests are made for chronically sick people, the blood is assessed for various chemical compounds and elements and a count is made of the red blood cells (erythrocytes) and white blood cells (leucocytes). A more thorough inspection of the blood under a microscope, however, reveals a lot more. Such an inspection of the blood of someone chronically ill shows that the blood is polluted with sludge and that the red cells and blood platelets tend to stick together (aggregate), so that the blood becomes sticky (high viscosity); it cannot carry oxygen properly and it cannot circulate properly. This, of course, is a demonstration of a diseased *milieu interieur*, reflected in medical tests by increased blood pressure, high sedimentation rate of red cells (ESR) and high platelet adhesion index (PAI).

It is common knowledge among doctors that these poor blood conditions accompany the various chronic diseases, but their conventional drug-oriented medical training does not permit them to see that the impure, high viscosity, sludged blood is the disease itself, and that what they think is the disease is only a symptom of disturbed homeostasis.

When it is suspected that an unidentified illness may be caused by a germ or virus and a more highly powered microscopic inspection of the blood is made, confusion again arises because of the many forms of microbes displayed and because the forms do not always remain constant (see Chapter 5). The more the blood deteriorates, the greater the number of microbes present, which multiply not as the cause of the illness, but as a result of it. One way or another, a patient receiving medical treatment is assured of one thing—he will not go short of antibiotics and other drugs until he either escapes the system or is finally and expensively "cured" to death, when the initial problem was really toxemia and lost homeostasis.

Although medical drugs may sometimes provide relief from disease symptoms, in the long run they cannot do anything but harm to the patient because, as unnatural substances in the body, they place further strain on already overworked organs which correctly sense a drug to be a poison to be neutralized and expelled. Thus drugs only cause further deterioration of the *milieu interieur* with consequential additional distress, the symptoms of which are nonchalantly referred to as "side effects". When, as often happens, additional medicine is prescribed to counter the side effects, the vicious circle is complete. Thus it is easy to understand why iatrogenic disease[1] is now recognized as a major cause of death, which of course it always has been.

Many intelligent doctors, after realizing the absurdity of allopathic medical methods, have abandoned their old beliefs in medicines and drugs and become medical heretics, which of course brings them disfavor in orthodox medical circles and no chance to present their newfound beliefs in professional journals. Therefore many such experienced doctors write books[2] to present their information direct to the populace. Two such doctors are Hans Selye, author of *The Stress of Life*, and Reino Virtonen, author of *Claude Bernard and Experimental Medicine*. These books are mentioned here because they both quote Louis Pasteur, father of the Germ Theory of Disease, who, just before his death in 1895, said to his friend Professor Renon: "Bernard was right, the germ is nothing, the milieu is everything."

---

[1] Disease caused by medical treatment.

[2] Refer to the book list in the Appendix.

CHAPTER 3

Toxemia and the Diseases of Civilization

I know of nothing so potent in maintaining good health in laboratory animals as perfectly constituted food; I know of nothing so potent in producing ill-health as improperly constituted food. This, too, is the experience of stock breeders. Is man an exception to a rule so universally applicable to the higher animals?

Major General Sir Robert McCarrison,
CIE MD D.Sc LL.D FRCP

Toxemia is a polluted condition of the body's *milieu interieur*, due to impurities in the bloodstream derived from improperly constituted food and to a lesser extent from other sources.

The diseases of civilization in some cases commence before birth due to malnutrition and toxemia of the mother in pregnancy. From birth onwards they appear in a fairly predictable sequence in the average person and are so common they are generally assumed to be a more or less normal part of human existence. The sequence starts with various minor respiratory infections, proceeding to tooth decay, occasional flu, acne, dandruff, constipation and so on, all considered quite to be expected. As people grow older the more troublesome problems appear, such as premenstrual tension and headaches in women, slowly increasing blood pressure, the need for reading glasses, back problems and so forth. From this stage it is only a short step to arthritis, diabetes, circulatory and digestive problems, ulcers, gallstones, kidney stones, bowel problems, glaucoma, and finally cataracts, prostate disorders, osteoporosis, senility, Alzheimer's disease—if heart attack, stroke or cancer have not already broken the sequence. These are only the common ones, but common or uncommon they are all malfunctions caused by toxemia; they are symptoms of toxemia. Toxemia is the real disease.

The different manifestations of disease, being of mainly dietary origin, vary according to the nature of the dietary faults responsible, and thus different countries and communities display varying disease patterns which differ according to the traditional diets and other living habits which are followed. Whereas, in the Western nations, there was once a distinction between the so-called diseases of affluence and the deficiency diseases common among the poor, today that distinction has just about disappeared due to the improved financial situation of the lower classes, so that now just about everybody can enjoy the pleasures of the "supermarket" Western diet and suffer the diseases of affluence together.

In brief:

Toxemia	=	impurities and deficiencies of the blood (see "Mineral Deficiencies" in Chapter 14).
Disease	=	dysfunction of normal body processes.
Civilization	=	society of developed culture, art and science.

Why humans get sick and wild animals do not formula: The art of cooking + the science of chemistry and medicine = toxemia and the diseases of civilization.

Improperly constituted food—to use Dr McCarrison's expression—although life sustaining, is at the same time health destroying because it does not furnish the life-sustaining components in the proper form or quantity, and in addition introduces, directly or indirectly, toxic substances into the bloodstream. Thus the digestive system is constantly overworked and the *milieu interieur* is constantly in a state of toxemia, the degree of which is dependent on the vitality of the eliminatory organs. The manner in which the body is impaired and the symptoms of impairment displayed are dependent on the degree and nature of the toxemia.

Because there are countless variations in the nature and degree of toxemia, there are countless variations in symptoms, which accounts for why there are so many diseases doctors must try to remember the names of in their mistaken belief that each symptom represents a different disease.

All races of people are sickness prone, some to a greater or lesser extent than others, for the simple reason that humans everywhere tamper one way or another with natural food—mostly by cooking—and often consume food not really suited to their systems at all, in addition to which they practise other harmful habits.

The traditional Western diet—that is, one high in fat, protein, cholesterol, salt, sugar, condiments and so on—contains plenty of nutrients, but in the wrong proportions, too much of it cooked, and too much of it altogether. That the Western diet can sustain health is a fact, but it does so only if the digestive system can perform the difficult task of breaking it down and assimilating it while at the same time effectively disposing of the toxic by-products produced. Thus no matter what the diet, the duration of healthy years and the ultimate duration of life depends on how long the integrity of the body's vital organs can be maintained under whatever strain they may be forced to endure. All forms of animal life respond to unnatural food in the same way. Horses fed on oats and chaff will maintain reasonable health and live for twenty-five years, but on good natural pastures will maintain better health and live for fifty years. Similarly, dogs and cats fed only on canned and packaged foods never display best condition nor live as long as those fed exclusively on raw meat.[1]

Toxins are produced in the body from the best of diets as natural by-products of normal metabolism and are eliminated effortlessly by the organs of elimination without the slightest wear and tear. The toxins that do all the harm leading to premature degeneration and disease are the toxins resultant from eating the wrong food. These toxins are not the chemicals from additives and poison sprays, etc that are in the food to start with, but they are actually

---

[1] An example of how imperfectly constituted food eaten by a mother in pregnancy and beforehand can cause physical and mental deformities in the offspring is given from the cat feeding experiments of Francis M. Pottenger, MD, of California. Dr Pottenger conducted experiments involving 900 cats over a ten-year period from 1932–42, having noticed how dietary deficiencies constantly occurred in experimental animals fed on a scientifically formulated, supposedly perfectly constituted diet which contained some cooked food.

On a diet of raw meat and pasteurized milk or on a diet of cooked meat and raw milk, the cats' health deteriorated, whereas cats fed on raw meat and raw milk maintained perfect condition. The offspring of the ailing cats were weak and deformed with slack or perverted interest in sex, and those that survived to adulthood and were capable of breeding produced either stillborn or pathetically weak kittens. There were no further generations of the weakened cats because this generation was incapable of even attempting to breed.

When such cats of the second generation were put on the raw diet, their health improved and breeding from them was successful. However, Dr Pottenger reported that even properly fed, it took four further generations of this group before the line became completely normal again.

Pottenger recorded that when cats were fed raw milk from dry feed cows instead of raw milk from fresh feed cows, they showed deterioration similar to cats fed pasteurized milk. (See *Pottenger's Cats, A Study in Nutrition*, Price Pottenger Foundation, La Mesa, California.)

produced within the body as by-products of the body's efforts to produce pure nourishment from impure materials. While man-made chemicals in food are undesirable and probably harmful to some extent, so little harm do they cause compared to body-produced toxemia that it is a pointless exercise to be concerned about them without first removing the main factors.

The toxins which are products of normal metabolism arise from two sources:

1 The unwanted by-products of digestive functions which from natural food are of low potency and easily expelled via the kidneys and urine.
2 The waste products of the body's cells which are carried away in the lymph fluid and bloodstream to be expelled via the kidneys (urine), the lungs (carbon dioxide) and the skin (sweat).

The abnormal toxins which cause disease when they overload the liver and kidneys and pollute the blood and *milieu interieur* are:

1 The unwanted by-products of digestive functions (as in 1 above), except in greater quantity and higher potency due to the more complicated molecular structure of cooked food, excess protein, etc.
2 Incompletely digested substances entering the blood-stream direct from the digestive tract such as fat particles, cholesterol, protein molecules, salt, condiments, etc, which not only cause toxemia but, by making the blood sticky, impede its circulation.
3 Toxins from infected teeth; mercury from amalgam fillings.
4 Chemicals contained in food, liquor, smoke and water (fluoride and chlorine at the levels commonly used in public water supplies are toxic and immuno-supressive, as are minerals such as copper and lead from pipes or bore water).
5 Medicine and drugs of any kind.
6 Stress-induced hormonal chemicals.

7 Last, and probably the most harmful—various acids and toxins produced in the colon by bacterial putrification of improperly digested remnants of cooked, high-fat, high-protein food which enter the bloodstream in the water reabsorbed from the colon back into the circulation.

It can be seen then, that depending mainly on the sort of food eaten from day to day, toxemia within the body can vary over short periods of time from normal safe levels to levels high enough to disrupt bodily functions in many different ways, wearing out its organs and eventually causing death by functional breakdown of the body's life processes. Thus the quality of life and length of its duration may range from zero to perhaps 120 years according to the degree to which toxemia is allowed to exist in the *milieu interieur* of the body.

The healthiest and longest-lived people in the world are accepted generally to be the Hunzas of northern Pakistan and the people in the Caucasus of Russia, whereas the shortest-lived are the Eskimos and Lapplanders of the Arctic. Sir Robert McCarrison, Major General, Indian Medical Service, described the Hunzas thus:

> The diet of these people corresponds in many ways to that of the Sikhs; but they eat less meat, and, their stocks being limited to goats, their consumption of milk and milk products is less than that of the Sikhs. But they are great fruit-eaters, especially of apricots and mulberries, which they use in both the raw and sun-dried state. The power of endurance of these people is extraordinary: to see a man of this race throw off his scanty garments, revealing a figure which would delight the eye of a Rodin, and plunge into a glacier-fed river in the middle of winter with as much unconcern as many of us would take a tepid bath, is to realize that perfection of physique and great physical endurance are attainable on the simplest of foods, providing these be of the right kind. These people are long-lived and vigorous in old age. Among them, the

ailments so common in our own people—such as gastro-intestinal disorders, colitis, gastro and duodenal ulcer and cancer—are extraordinarily uncommon, and I have no doubt whatever in my own mind that their freedom from these scourges of modern civilization is due to three things:

1. Their use of simple, natural foodstuffs of the right kind;
2. Their vigorous outdoor life; and
3. Their fine bracing climate.

With the Hunzas resistance to infection is remarkable . . . gastro-intestinal complaints, dyspepsia, ulcers, colitis, and appendicitis are at least as uncommon as they are common elsewhere. Cancer is so rare that in nine years' practice I never came across a single case of it.

The Eskimos[2] by comparison rated this description by Dr Samuel Hutton, who observed them over the period 1902 to 1913, from his book *Health Conditions and Disease Incidence Among the Eskimos of Labrador*:

> Old age sets in at fifty and its signs are strongly marked at sixty. In the years beyond sixty the Eskimo is aged and feeble. Comparatively few live beyond sixty and only a very few reach seventy. Those who live to such an age have spent a life of great activity, feeding on Eskimo foods and engaging in characteristically Eskimo pursuits . . . Careful records have been left by the missionaries for more than a hundred years.

It was also noted that the Eskimos had very low resistance to infectious diseases and suffered severe osteoporosis as they got older. A later study of a small

[2] The word Eskimo is derived from the language of the Cree Indians and means "eater of raw meat". It should be noted that the descriptions given of both the Hunzas and the Eskimos are those made early in the 20th Century before they began to discard their traditional and more primitive way of life.

population (about 1000) on the east coast of Greenland by Hoygaard and Pedersen, Copenhagen 1941, showed an average lifespan of only twenty-seven and a half years mainly due to premature degeneration of adults. Their diet was ninety-five per cent flesh food but it was not stated whether the Eskimos had adopted the white man's practice of cooking their food.

There is the comparison. Dr McCarrison attributed the excellence of the Hunzas to their diet, outdoor activity and bracing climate, so in view of the fact the Eskimos also indulged in much outdoor activity in a bracing climate, the distinction in their health status compared to the Hunzas is clearly due to dietary differences.

Now the dubious health standards of all "developed" countries are pretty similar to each other and the diseases of civilization occur among them in roughly the same proportions regardless of climate, and only a little influenced by occupation. Clearly diet is the problem, so let us look at a comparison of the typical American diet with that of the Hunzas.

These figures tell us that, on average, Americans consume over four times the amount of fat and twice the amount of protein than that consumed by a Hunza man while at the same time less carbohydrate, most of which is sugar or otherwise refined and fiberless.

Average Daily Intake (Grams)	Kilojoules (Calories)	Fats Gm		Protein Gm		Carbohydrates Gm	
Americans all ages	13,860 (3300)	157	40%	100	13%	380 Mostly refined	47%
Hunzas— adult males	8,080 (1923)	36	15%	50	10%	354 Mostly unrefined	75%

(Percentages indicate proportion of total kilojoules/calories)

These figures tell us why Americans (and the rest of us) experience weight problems and mediocre health and die of heart disease, cancer and the other diseases of civilisation.

Note: This comparison of the Hunza diet to the American diet is for comparison purposes only, and is not made to convey the impression that the Hunza diet is an optimum one (which it is not). For discussion on what constitutes an optimum diet see Chapter 14.

Protein and Fat as Causes of Toxemia

The main sources of protein and fat in the Western diet are of animal origin and thus contain cholesterol in quantities harmful to the human body. However, many pure vegetarians also suffer toxemia to a dangerous extent because their diet is based heavily on grain products and lentils, which are very high in vegetable protein, and in many cases include liberal quantities of concentrated vegetable oils.

The by-products of the metabolism of fat and protein which are potentially harmful are chemicals called ketones from fat, and uric acid and ammonia from protein. It is mainly these substances in excessive amounts which overtax the kidneys, sometimes to the extent of destroying them. For this reason it is wise for people on the traditional Western diet to drink copious quantities of water to flush out the kidneys. Not only do heavy protein-eaters need to urinate often, their urine is dark in color and odorous. Observers of primitive Eskimos in the early 1900s described how in winter the Eskimos had to go out into the freezing cold at frequent intervals to urinate and how they would return inside bringing snow to make more drinking water.

Apart from the toxins so produced, the condition of the bloodstream can be seriously degraded by particles of fat and cholesterol entering the bloodstream directly from the intestine via the lymph circulation, so much so at times that the blood appears milky red instead of crimson. In this situation the blood's red cells stick together in bunches called rouleaux, which block the fine capillary vessels and deprive the tissues of circulation, causing the tingling sensation of "pins and needles". At the same time the blood platelets also adhere to each other and the blood plasma itself becomes sticky, so up goes the blood pressure as the heart works harder. The white cells of the immune system become inhibited in function as well, and the entire scene becomes a set-up for disaster, disaster meaning every disease in the book. No wonder people lack vitality, need a lot of sleep, catch colds and get headaches, but these are only minor signs of the troubles that lie ahead if the toxemia is allowed to persist.

The most poisonous form of toxemia, however, originates in the colon (large bowel) because of constipation, which on the Western diet is unavoidable due to a lack of dietary fiber. It must be understood that a person can be "as regular as clockwork" and still be constipated. On a natural diet of mainly fruit and vegetables (raw), low in protein and fat, the indigestible cellulose remnants are quickly processed for elimination on reaching the colon by the normal aerobic bacteria there and are then readily defecated, having made the entire transit of the digestive tract in about twenty-four hours. However, when the undigested remnants of a high-fat, high-protein diet arrive in the colon they are difficult to break down further, and the normal aerobic bacteria must change in form to an anaerobic form which putrefies the remnants and produces different acids and toxic chemicals. Because meat, chicken, fish, dairy products and refined carbohydrates are completely lacking in fiber, the process is slow moving. Thus the "transit time" of the Western diet is about seventy-two hours instead of twenty-four, giving the potent toxins ample time to be absorbed into the body by way of the bile circulation and to set up the irritation which leads to appendicitis and bowel cancer.

A graphic illustration of how auto-intoxication from the colon causes all manner of disease is the experience of Sir William Arbuthnot Lane,[3] the famous English physician and surgeon. Sir William first realized that the bowel was the source of many health problems when, after surgically removing diseased bowels, he noted that his patients' health rapidly improved and various diseases such as arthritis, gall bladder "involvements", thyroid "difficulties", etc disappeared in a few days. At first his surgical training influenced him to specialize in removing peoples' colons, until it occurred to him from the biologist, Sir Arthur Keith's, studies of wild apes that the entire problem could be eliminated simply by dietary means.

That the problem of chemicals such as preservatives, coloring agents, etc in food is one of relatively minor importance compared to body-produced toxemia is illustrated in some interesting comparisons of disease incidence in different countries. Denmark has very strict prohibition against most food additives, while Norway and Sweden do not. Despite this, Denmark has a cancer incidence twenty per cent higher than Norway and Sweden,[4] which is explainable by the fact that Denmark per capita consumes twenty per cent more fat in the diet. But another comparison, this time between Denmark and Finland, showed that in relation to colon cancer, meat was a greater danger than fat, because the Finns consumed even more fat than the Danes but had only a quarter as much colon cancer. That Denmark suffers four times the bowel cancer rate of Finland is explainable only by the Danes' much heavier meat consumption (from the *International Agency for Research on Cancer 1977*).

When people speak of "cleansing diets", they mean diets which do not cause toxemia. Cleansing the *milieu interieur* is performed by the body itself, which of course it is trying to do all the time but can only accomplish properly when freed of constant overloads. The quickest way to achieve inner cleanliness is by not eating anything

---

[3] *The Prevention of The Diseases Peculiar to Civilization* by Sir William Arbuthnot Lane (1929).

[4] Cancer Research, Vol. 35, p. 3379, K. Carroll.

at all, ie fasting, and consuming water only for an indefinite period, but this requires tuition and supervision and will be discussed later. The role of garlic and other herbs in improving health when used therapeutically seems to be in emulsifying fat in the blood and lowering blood viscosity, but of course the real answer is not to put the fat in there in the first place.

In Western civilization it is well known that women on the average have a lifespan advantage of several years over men mainly because they are less prone to heart disease in their earlier years, but that after menopause they suffer vascular problems at the same rate as men. This protection enjoyed by women is obviously provided by a function males do not experience—menstruation, which is Nature's way of detoxifying a woman's body in preparation for an anticipated pregnancy. The degree of distress experienced in menstruation by some women is proportional to the degree of toxemia existing within them, and it is noteworthy that some women, who by virtue of superior diet are toxin free, suffer little or no discomfort or blood loss with their periods, as is also the case with fit women athletes whose body functions work more adequately to detoxify them all the time. Menstruation should therefore not be considered a 'curse' at all—it is a blessing that protects. It is the Western diet that is the curse. It is noteworthy, too, in relation to the superior health of the Hunzas, that there is also a difference in average life expectancy of about five years between males and females, which in this case favors the males who are by virtue of their occupations far more physically active than the women.

A disease which has not been recognized until recently but which has always been and is becoming still more common is iatrogenic disease, which means disease caused by medical treatment. Many sick people die of what are called "complications", and it is a fact that many such complications consist of metabolic malfunctions caused by medical drugs, all of which are depressants of the immune system. A less frightening example of iatrogenic disease is the frequency of various infections which appear to be contagious among hospital patients while at the same time the doctors and hospital staff remain unaffected.

Medical knowledge of the etiology (underlying causes) of most diseases is practically zero because the practice of medicine is founded on medieval beliefs in devils and potions, and it is significant that the wiser with age and experience a good doctor gets, the less he believes in the efficacy of his potions.

Most of the medicine prescribed by doctors they have little knowledge about other than the sales pitch given them by the pharmaceutical representatives (have you ever perused a medical journal?), but it is a pretty safe bet that if doctors ever studied the fine print in the drug manuals on the side effects of these drugs they would think twice before taking any themselves. It is also a pretty safe bet that if the patients ever got to read the fine print, they would quickly find the strength to run away.

Be that as it may, the main purpose of this chapter is to point out the mostly unsuspected dangers of auto-intoxication—toxemia generated within the body from our favorite foods—and to warn against the further toxemia produced in the body by the well-meaning efforts of the medical doctors who try to "cure" the effects of the first lot but only make it worse.

John H. Tilden, MD, said it all back in 1926. Summing up in his book *Toxemia Explained*:

> "In chronic disease, the treatment, first, last and all the time, must be with a view of getting rid of the toxemia. This consists of correcting whatever habits of life are producing enervation, and then gradually building up a normal digestion, assimilation and elimination.
>
> After fifty years of floundering in the great sea of medical and surgical speculation to find the causes of so-called diseases, all I could find was that all the people were sick part of the time, and part of the people were sick all of the time. But Glory be, all of the people were not sick all of the time.

Some people got well under my treatment and
friends would say that I 'cured' them. Others died,
and friends would say that Providence removed
them. I knew that I did not cure those who got
well, and I did not like to acknowledge even to
myself that I had killed those who died.

It took a long time to evolve out of the one
conventional idea of many diseases into the truth
that there is but ONE disease, and that the four
hundred catalogued so-called diseases are but
different manifestations of Toxemia—blood and
tissue uncleanliness.''

CHAPTER 4

The Immune System

For twenty-one years I was able to study the reaction of well-fed animals to epidemic diseases, such as rinderpest, foot-and-mouth disease, septicemia and so forth, which frequently devastated the countryside. None of my animals were segregated, none were inoculated; they frequently came in contact with diseased stock. No case of infectious disease occurred. The reward of well-nourished protoplasm was a very high degree of disease resistance, which might even be described as immunity.

Sir Albert Howard

The immune system is the name given to the complex organisation of glands, white cells, antibodies and other protein substances, hormones, enzymes and bacteria which protect the body against potentially harmful germs, viruses and foreign substances that may gain access to it. Foreign substances may include improperly digested protein molecules or other toxic matter from the digestive system as well as medicine and antibiotics also toxic to the body. The moment any of these substances enter the bloodstream they excite antagonism from the immune system and are therefore called antigens. Among the everyday activities of the white cells is the destruction and elimination of worn-out red blood cells, which are continually replaced by the millions every second, and the elimination of any other cellular or metabolic debris.

White cells are called leucocytes and there are many types, each with a different way of working but co-operating together as circumstances require to achieve their joint purpose. White cells are constantly being manufactured in the bone marrow of the body and migrate to inhabit all the tissues and body fluids in great numbers, whereas red blood cells (erythrocytes) never leave the blood circulation.

Phagocytes are white cells which destroy antigens by consuming and digesting them. Macrophages are large phagocytes which can consume larger antigens such as defective or worn-out body cells. Neutrophils are the most numerous of the mobile phagocytes and are primarily concerned in attending to foreign germs or viruses. Lymphocytes are another type of white cell which patrol in the blood and lymph, there being two kinds: B lymphocytes, which manufacture antibodies, and T lymphocytes, which have other specialized functions for which they have been prepared in the thymus gland. Antibodies are specialised protein substances which B lymphocytes produce in large numbers when necessary to help destroy an antigen of a particular kind. The antibodies are so specialized they will be effective only against one particular antigen, so even after the antigen has been destroyed, tests of the specific antibody retained in the body for possible future use will allow identification of the antigen for which the antibody was made. Thus a blood test which discloses the presence of a certain antibody may indicate either the presence of its associated antigen (such as a virus) or that it has been present but now destroyed.

T lymphocytes are so named because they are special products of the thymus gland, and it is from the observations of T cells that the condition of the immune system can be assessed, as for instance in AIDS. Another indicator of immune potential is the total number of white cells in a cubic millimetre of blood, normal being considered 5000 to 7000, perhaps as high as 10,000, this higher figure being an indication of a toxic system. It is normal for numbers to increase with activity, stress or challenge by antigens, but sometimes greatly increased numbers will indicate toxicity tending towards leukemia.

Inflammation and fever are another response of the

immune system and may occur locally at an area of infection or as the raised temperature of the entire body. As all vital functions in the body are brought about by enzyme activity, and as enzyme activity is greatly increased with increased temperature, fever which accompanies infection is an indication of good immune response. Often accompanying infection is swelling and soreness of the lymph glands nearest the seat of infection and this is an indication that the immune system is attempting to contain the infection where it is.

The capability of the immune system (immuno-competence) depends on the general state of health and physical fitness, but regardless of this may be drastically (but only temporarily) reduced in a healthy body by fatigue or excessive stress. The condition of the bloodstream is very important. When toxemia exists, and fat in the blood tends to stick blood cells and platelets into sludge, increasing blood viscosity and decreasing oxygen levels, the immune system along with the rest of the entire body becomes severely diminished in function. Thus various chronic disease conditions, such as cancer, are invariably marked by diminished vitality, low body temperature, low enzyme levels and low immunocompetence. Chronically ill people and senile people, therefore, more readily succumb to acute infection.

In particular, the level of immunocompetence depends on a healthy thymus, which in concert with the other endocrine glands directs the activities of the immune system. When health fails, or excessive demand is made on the immune system by way of infection or mental or physical trauma, the thymus, overworked, becomes exhausted, shrinks in size and loses function. Physical trauma includes toxemia, a great deal of which is produced within the body from wrong food, as previously described. Contributing to toxemia, however, are a great number of other substances harmful to the body and its immune system such as all drugs, medicinal or otherwise, antibiotics (refer to "AIDS" in Chapter 7), tranquillizers, pain killers, aspirin and so on, nicotine, marijuana, exhaust fumes, fluoride and chlorine, etc in water supplies. And to repeat, it is a fact that mental trauma alone, such as the pronouncement of cancer or AIDS, is capable of sealing a sick person's fate in a fashion like that of the bone pointing ritual of Aboriginals or the decree of death by a tribal witchdoctor.

An illustration of how mental trauma diminishes the immune system is given by Dr Laurence E. Badgley of San Francisco in his books *Choose To Live* and *Healing AIDS Naturally:*

"T4 white blood cell counts are intimately related to mental focus. One of my patients was without symptoms and went to another doctor for an AIDS test. The doctor did the test, which was positive, as well as the T4 helper cell count which was 494 and normal. Upon learning that his antibody test was positive, the patient went into a tailspin of depression and fear. One week later he returned to the doctor because of his anxiety, and his T4 helper cell count was taken again. After one week of depression and no other symptoms his T4 count fell over 50% to 234.

This intimate relationship of the mind and body raises a question about the true nature of the AIDS epidemic. It is not far fetched to postulate that much of the immune system depression among AIDS-test-positive patients might be the result of doctors telling them that it is likely they will get AIDS and die. The brain is a giant immune system gland that operates on hope, joy, and optimism. The gland turns off in response to mental attitudes of fear and depression.

The question is raised as to how many people are dying because they have been programmed to die. The observation is made that doctors who tell their patients they have a terminal disease are programming their patients to die. The charge is made that these doctors are performing malpractise."

Thus to obtain the best chances for a patient's recovery it behoves a doctor to not only avoid programming his patient negatively, but to go further and program the patient positively by encouraging optimism, hope and confidence. It is the capability to do this that allows some doctors to constantly achieve better results than others.

All vitamins and minerals[1] are important for proper immune function, particularly vitamin C, and the generally inadequate amount of this vitamin in the Western diet, together with excessive quantities of fat, cholesterol and protein, are two of the main reasons for the mediocre standard of immunocompetence displayed by most people. A recent report in the *Cecil Textbook of Medicine* stated that sixty per cent of all human illness occurs in the upper respiratory tract in the form of colds, influenza and secondary bacterial infections. The survey showed an average of 5.6 infections per adult per year. Whereas a fit and healthy person is resistant to all infections and in ordinary circumstances suffers no respiratory problems at all year in year out, the 5.6 average shows that the average standard of immunocompetence is disturbingly poor. However, by comparison, our general standard of immuno-competence is superior compared with that of some other countries, but this proves only that the people in those countries are sicker than we are. In some countries where the majority of people are underfed and malnourished all the time, epidemics occur frequently, and history reveals that epidemics were often consequential in the wake of wars or natural disasters when shortage of fresh food resulted in widespread malnutrition. Such epidemics occur not because germs and viruses automatically increase in numbers during wars and floods; they occur because malnutrition weakens the people and reduces their powers of resistance.

Whereas there are people in the world such as the Hunzas, who as a race maintain better health and greater

[1] *See* "Mineral Deficiencies", Chapter 14.

resistance to disease than we do, they are by no means perfect specimens. Perfect specimens are only to be found in environments perfectly suited to them where the food perfectly suited to them is plentiful and not altered from its natural state. Thus the only perfect specimens to be found in the world are wild animals. While their natural food is plentiful, wild animals never get respiratory infections, tooth decay, skin complaints, venereal diseases and so on because they lack the skills to "improve" their food and otherwise complicate their lives. Their immune systems are not one scrap better than human immune systems—they are to all intents and purposes exactly the same—it's just that their immune systems are fully functional while human immune systems are always to a greater or lesser extent handicapped by toxemia and stress. Animals, too, can in this way be handicapped and thereby suffer infections, but investigation shows that these are always animals domesticated or confined by man and fed unnatural food. The most common examples of this are pet dogs and cats fed on "perfectly balanced" canned and packaged foods. These animals not only get sick from time to time, have tablets and injections, but even get heart disease and cancer. Perhaps the best example of both impaired and unimpaired immunocompetence in animals is the comparison between the cattle managed by Sir Albert Howard and the cattle of neighboring farmers where Sir Albert's herds at times mixed freely with others suffering foot and mouth disease, etc without ever getting sick.

It's pretty simple—look after your immune system and it will look after you. It is immensely powerful in sound health but it becomes diminished in many people because of the many challenges it receives, challenges for which it was not designed.

Immunization

The intention of medical vaccinations is to artificially induce the body's immune system into producing antibodies to microbes of various diseases so that if at some later time the microbe (or virus) is encountered in reality, the immune system will be forearmed. The method is to make a vaccine from a deactivated form of the microbe which, when injected, is harmless to the body but capable of producing the desired reaction to achieve immunity.

The theory of immunization is based on the germ theory of disease, and like the germ theory it has caused a great deal of confusion because it is full of inconsistencies, failing more often than when it appears to work. Too often adverse reactions occur after vaccinations, and the record shows that over the years more suffering and deaths have eventuated from immunization than would have occurred without it.

Since Edward Jenner demonstrated the use of cowpox vaccine against smallpox in 1796, vaccinations against smallpox were started. Despite this, a smallpox epidemic swept England in 1839 and killed 22,081 people. In 1853 the Government made smallpox vaccinations compulsory, but the incidence of the disease kept increasing, and in 1872 another epidemic killed 44,840 people, most of whom were vaccinated. The compulsory vaccination law was abolished in 1948. Similar disasters occurred in Germany and Japan, but possibly the worst was in the Philippines in 1918 when the US Government forced over three million natives to be vaccinated. Of these, 47,369 came down with smallpox and 16,477 died. In 1919 the program was doubled, and over seven million were vaccinated, of whom 65,180 came down with the disease and 44,408 died. The epidemic was a direct result of the vaccination program. These facts are described by Dr William F. Koch in his book *The Survival Factor in Neoplastic and Viral Disease* (1961). Dr Koch further described the disastrous increase in polio incidence in the USA and Canada following the mass inoculation campaign against polio in 1958. The highest increase was 700 per cent in Ottowa, Canada. Dr Robert Mendelsohn in his book *Confessions of a Medical Heretic* questions the safety of all immunizations, including diphtheria and whooping cough, in a chapter titled, "If this is Preventive Medicine, I'll Take My Chances with Disease!"

Richard Moskowitz, MD, of New York in his lecture "Immunizations—A Dissenting View"[2] commenced by saying:

> "For the past 10 years or so, I have felt a deep and growing compunction against giving routine immunizations to children. It began with the fundamental belief that people have the right to make that choice for themselves. Soon I discovered that I could no longer bring myself to give the injections even when the parents wished me to.
>
> At bottom, I have always felt that the attempt to eradicate entire microbial species from the biosphere must inevitably upset the balance of nature in fundamental ways that we can as yet scarcely imagine. Such concerns loom ever larger as new vaccines continue to be developed, seemingly for no better reason than that we have the technical capacity to make them and thereby to demonstrate our power, as a civilization, to manipulate the evolutionary process itself.
>
> Purely from the viewpoint of our own species, even if we could be sure that the vaccines were harmless, the fact remains that they are compulsory [in many states of the USA], that all children are required to undergo them without any sensitive regard for basic differences in individual

---

[2] From the book *Dissent in Medicine, Nine Doctors Speak Out* (on the issues of How Much Science is there in Modern Medicine?; Corruption in American Medicine; The Inaccuracies of Medical Testing; Hospital Births; Immunizations; Cancer Treatment; and Environmental Issues), Robert S. Mendelsohn, MD, George Crile, MD, Samuel Epstein, MD, Henry Heimlich, MD, Alan Scott Levin, MD, Edward R. Pinckney, MD, David Spodick, MD, Richard Moskowitz, MD, George White, MD, Contemporary Books, Chicago 1985.

susceptibility, to say nothing of the wishes of the parents or the children themselves.

Most people can readily accept the fact that, from time to time, certain laws that some of us strongly disagree with may be necessary for the public good. But the issue in this case involves nothing less than the introduction of foreign proteins or even live viruses into the bloodstream of entire populations. For that reason alone, the public is surely entitled to convincing proof, beyond any reasonable doubt, that artificial immunization is in fact a safe and effective procedure, in no way injurious to health, and that the threat of the corresponding natural diseases remains sufficiently clear and urgent to warrant mass inoculation of everyone, even against their will if necessary.

Unfortunately, such proof has never been given; and, even if it could be, continuing to employ vaccines against diseases that are no longer prevalent or no longer dangerous hardly qualifies as an emergency.

Finally, even if such an emergency did exist, and artificial immunization could be shown to be an appropriate response to it, the decision would remain essentially a *political* one, involving issues of public health and safety that are far too important to be settled by any purely scientific or technical criteria, or indeed by *any* criteria less authoritative than the clearly articulated sense of the community about to be subjected to it.

For all of these reasons, I want to present the case against routine immunization as clearly and forcefully as I can. What I have to say is not quite a formal theory capable of rigorous proof or disproof. It is simply an attempt to explain my own experience, a nexus of interrelated facts, observations, reflections and hypotheses.

I offer them to the public in part because the growing refusal of parents to vaccinate their children is so seldom articulated or taken seriously. The fact is that we have been taught to accept vaccination as a sort of involuntary communion, a sacrament of our own participation in the unrestricted growth of scientific and industrial technology, utterly heedless of the long-term consequences to the health of our own species, let alone to the balance of nature as a whole. For that reason alone, the other side of the case urgently needs to be heard."

Dr Moskowitz went on to describe how the incidence of whooping cough had already precipitously declined long before the pertussis vaccine was introduced, as had tuberculosis, cholera, typhoid and other scourges of a bygone era similarly declined in response to better living conditions long before vaccines for them were developed, but that medical science had been mistakenly given credit for the improvement.

Dr Moskowitz's thirty years of observations of the sheer ineffectiveness of immunization programs makes one wonder why the procedures continue to be persevered with, but worse than the ineffectiveness are the severe and sometimes fatal reactions that frequently follow vaccinations, to an extent so bad that in many countries vaccination programs have been abandoned, while at the same time the World Health Organization (WHO) no longer insists that international travellers be vaccinated against the diseases once considered so dangerous. Dr Moskowitz said:

"Far from producing a genuine immunity, then, the vaccines may act by actually interfering with or *suppressing* the immune response as a whole, in much the same way that radiation, chemotherapy, and corticosteroids and other anti-inflammatory drugs do. Artificial immunization focuses on *antibody production*, a single aspect of the immune process, and disarticulates it and allows it to stand for the whole, in much the same way as chemical suppression of an elevated blood pressure is accepted as a valid substitute for a genuine *cure* of the patient whose blood pressure has risen. Worst of all, by making it difficult or impossible to mount a vigorous, acute response to infection, artificial immunization substitutes for it a much weaker, *chronic* response with little or no tendency to heal itself spontaneously."

That the sudden introduction of a foreign substance into the tissues of the body is sensed by the body as a traumatic event is easily comprehensible, particularly when the body is that of a tiny infant, and it is little wonder that the vaccinations of infants is held to be by many doctors the prime factor in infant cot deaths. (Refer to *Second Thoughts About Disease* by Doctors Archie Kalokerinos and Glen Dettman 1977, and *Vaccinations Condemned*, Better Life Research, 1981.)

Dr Moskowitz considered all vaccinations distinctly dangerous, particularly the administration to infants of the pertussis vaccine (whooping cough), a procedure now abandoned in Germany, in regard to which he says:

"Pertussis is also extremely variable clinically, ranging in severity from asymptomatic, mild, or inapparent infections, which are quite common actually, to very rare cases in young infants less than five months of age, in which the mortality is said to reach 40 percent. Indeed, the disease is rarely fatal or even that serious in children over a year old, and antibiotics have very little to do with the outcome.

A good deal of the pressure to immunize at the present time thus seems to be attributable to the higher death rate in very young infants, which has led to the terrifying practice of giving this most clearly dangerous of the vaccines to infants at two months of age, when their mother's milk would normally have protected them from all infections about as well as it can ever be done, and the effect

on the still developing blood and nervous system
could be catastrophic.

For all of these reasons, the practice of routine
pertussis immunization should be discontinued as
quickly as possible and more studies done to assess
and compensate the damage that it has already
done."

Pointing out that no proper studies have been ever
done on the effects of vaccinations, and that all the available
evidence shows them to be counter-productive, if not
outright dangerous, Dr Moskowitz concluded:

"In any case, the whole matter is clearly one of
enormous complexity, and illustrates only too well
the hidden dangers and miscalculations that are
inherent in the virtually irresistible attempt to beat
nature at her own game, to eliminate a problem
that cannot be eliminated, ie the *susceptibility* to
disease itself.

So even in the case of the polio vaccine, which
appears to be about as safe as any vaccine ever *can*
be, the same fundamental dilemma remains.
Perhaps the day will come when we can face the
consequences of deliberately feeding live
polioviruses to every living infant, and admit that
we should have left well enough alone, and
addressed ourselves to the art of healing the sick
when we have to, rather than to the technology of
eradicating the *possibility* of sickness, when we
don't have to, and can't possibly succeed in any
case."

Immunotherapy

Immunotherapy is the attempt to influence the course of
a disease by artificial manipulation of the immune system
after the disease has become established. Vaccines made
from blood samples, urine, etc have been used against a
number of diseases in an endeavor to stimulate a specific

immune response, as well as various other vaccines designed to stimulate the non-specific response. Results have always been disappointing, and this is no wonder.

Failure of immunotherapy is inevitable, because it is designed to stimulate artificially something which is exhausted. The solution is simple: forget about the immune system, forget about the tumor, headache, or what have you, and set about restoring the general health with diet, rest, relaxation, sunshine and exercise. The immune system will thereupon regenerate along with the rest of the body, thankful to be free of medical "help".

SUMMARIZING ON THE IMMUNE SYSTEM

It is barely recognized, but nevertheless true, that animals and plants, as well as men, can live peacefully with their most notorious microbial enemies. The world is obsessed by the fact that poliomyelitis can kill and maim several thousand unfortunate victims every year. But more extraordinary is the fact that millions upon millions of young people become infected by polio viruses, yet suffer no harm from the infection. The dramatic episodes of conflict between men and microbes are what strike the mind. What is less readily apprehended is the more common fact that infection can occur without producing disease.

Rene Dubos, Microbiologist
(*Mirage of Health*, Harper, 1959)

To a member of modern society, the "suffering no harm" that Dubos mentions appears extraordinary, but as he goes on to say, it is the more common fact. In a community properly endowed with health, the extraordinary event would be anybody getting sick at all.

To summarize the immune system:

- The capability of the immune system, when functioning properly, is far greater than generally imagined.

- The general level of health in civilized society is marginal, and therefore so too is the general level of immuno-competence.
- This accounts for the generally accepted high incidence of all kinds of infections, particularly influenza, and the increase in VD, herpes, hepatitis, candida and so on.
- Also associated with marginal health and poor immuno-competence is the relentless increase in cancer.
- The immune system cannot be artificially boosted; all it needs is a supply of decent blood with plenty of oxygen in a body free of stress and it soon regenerates of its own accord.

Factors that Affect the Immune System

Good:
Natural diet, happiness and serenity, high morale, a positive attitude, adequate rest and sleep, fresh air, physical exercise.

Adverse:
Most common
- toxemia from dietary errors, constipation;
- dietary deficiencies, in particular Vitamin C;
- worry;
- chemicals from different sources including fluoride, chlorine, etc in water supplies, pesticide residues in food, other chemicals in food; and
- medicine—aspirin, tranquillizers, cough mixtures, etc.

More severe
- alcohol;
- smoking;
- overweight;
- overwork, fatigue;
- mental trauma—anger, pain, worry, frustration, grief, fear;
- physical trauma—sexual excesses, excessive athletic training, prolonged discomfort, heat, cold; and

- chemical trauma—mercury in amalgam tooth fillings, poisons from infected teeth, poisons from insect bites, ticks, etc, septicemia, common medicines, prescription medicines, antibiotics, vaccinations.

Very severe
- severe malnutrition—junk food, high sugar, high salt, high fat, high cholesterol, severe vitamin C deficiency;
- all drugs used habitually whether taken intravenously, orally or inhaled, including marijuana, etc and antibiotics (refer to "AIDS" in Chapter 7);
- constant sexual promiscuity (*see* "AIDS");
- receptive anal sex (*see* "AIDS");
- bereavement, low self-esteem, guilt, hopelessness (*see* "AIDS"); and
- mental trauma of voodoo or bone-pointing death sentence by shaman, witchdoctor, or modern physician (*see* "AIDS").

CHAPTER 5

Germs and Viruses

For three centuries bacteria have been considered to be alien and awe inspiring, even by sophisticated professors and dedicated students. Most of us still think that these tiny living beings are primarily germs and pathogens. They are often named by the symptoms they (sometimes) cause: the syphilitic spirochete, the plague bacterium, the cholera vibrio and Legionella. In this book, Dr Sorin Sonea and his late colleague Dr Maurice Panisset, have begun to set the record straight. These organisms are not only our own ancestors but also are the basis of our life-support system. They supply our atmospheric gases, they cleanse our water supply, and, in general, they ensure us a livable environment.

Lyn Margulis, Professor of Biology,
Boston University;
from her Foreword to *A New Bacteriology* (1980)

All our lives we have been taught that germs are bad, that they are out to harm us. So we bathe daily using plenty of soap, wash our hands constantly and would never think of eating a food morsel picked up from the floor. We give the food morsel instead to the dog, which quickly gulps it down, hoping we will drop some more. But dogs, generally, stay in better health than people; some of the most fastidious people get sick quite often. Maybe there are more important things than germs and viruses to be concerned about; maybe we have the wrong idea about germs.

The principles of human survival are simple enough

but because it seems to be human nature to suspect anything simple, we have managed to weave so many complicated theories about human disease, human nutrition and the unique attraction humans have for germs and viruses that we cannot see the forest for the trees. Physiologically, humans are not unique at all, and but for the lifestyle errors they have themselves invented they would have no more reason to fear germs than a scruffy dog gnawing at a dirty old bone.

To understand better the natural relationship between germs and viruses and other forms of life, we must examine the fundamental principles that govern all forms of life on Earth. The first principle is that of symbiosis or co-existence, which states that all forms of life are one way or another dependent on each other, together forming what is known as the "web of life".

Of all forms of life on Earth, the vast majority are too small to be seen with the naked eye, inhabiting every minute space in the soil, water and atmosphere and on and within all larger creatures, and it was from such lowly forms of life that the higher forms evolved and upon which today the higher forms depend completely for their continued existence.

To believe in the evolution of the species doesn't mean you have to be an atheist, nor does it mean you have to accept word for word Charles Darwin's theory. That the higher species evolved from more primitive ones had been evident and speculated upon for centuries, and before Charles was born, his grandfather, Erasmus Darwin, respected doctor, inventor, poet and writer, himself had written a thesis on the subject.

Charles Darwin's theory of evolution was new only in that it presented a plausible explanation of the evolutionary process based on observed phenomena and not too much on imagination. Darwin did not invent the theory of evolution, he invented a theory of how it worked. Darwin believed, at least when his theory was published, that the changes in a species from one generation to another which led eventually to a new species altogether were entirely accidental, random changes, and that such random changes only became permanent if they conveyed an advantage giving a better chance of survival. He called this process "natural selection", and from this concept arose the expression "survival of the fittest".

Darwin's theory evolved in his mind from his observations as a naturalist, and his concept of natural selection is not in dispute. The part of his theory which has always been disputed is the belief that the evolutionary changes are random, occurring entirely by chance.

When the complexity of a single living cell is contemplated, it is inconceivable that random chance events in the wide open spaces—or for that matter, intelligently directed events in a modern laboratory—could ever have produced such an exquisitely complex thing. And even given a complete living cell to start with, and unlimited time, the number of random mutations needed to produce even something as lowly as an earthworm is so infinitely great that for them to occur with the necessary precision and exact sequence by sheer accident is beyond the remotest possibility. A humorous cartoon the author has never forgotten seeing in a color magazine years ago depicts an artist painting a portrait. Disgusted that he cannot get it right, the artist throws all his different colored paints into a bucket and hurls it all at the canvas. Then, looking back over his shoulder as he packs up his things to leave, he is suddenly transfixed. His eyes pop out. There smiling at him from the canvas, arms folded, in all her perfection, is—the Mona Lisa!

If then the supposition is correct that evolution could not occur by chance alone, it must be that there exists in Nature some guiding force which, even if working by trial and error, nevertheless works with a purpose. This was the conclusion arrived at by Darwin himself in his later years when speculating on the intricate structure of the human eye. Louis Pasteur was not the only scientist to have second thoughts on an unproven theory. Thus we talk about "the wisdom of Nature" and of "Nature's grand design", or simply acknowledge God Almighty. Who was it[1] said: "If God did not exist it would be necessary for man to invent him."? Thus it becomes clear that an understanding of evolution does not deny the existence of God; on the contrary, it confirms it.

When people talk about human evolution they usually assume it commenced only a few million years ago, starting from an ancestor in the form of some sort of ape. Others refer further back to the origin of the line of primates from which the apes evolved. But going even this far back reveals only changes in shape, size and brain capacity. Biologically and anatomically, the modern human is practically identical to these relatively immediate ancestors. So further and further back you can follow the evolutionary trail—granted with gaps here and there—and find that even earthworms have hearts, blood and immune systems of a rudimentary kind.

Did evolution start then with the first cell as many evolutionists suppose? How far back can we go? Well, if you really want to get involved, you can go back a long way further, because within every cell are contained living components and systems of greater complexity than ever, and research has shown that from the first appearance of life on Earth, it took several billion years for the aerobic cell itself to evolve, whereas all the rest since has taken but a billion years. In evolutionary terms the functioning cell was the breakthrough from which Nature could make trees and animals of all kinds. And finally (but hopefully not too finally) that dubious product, *Homo sapiens* . . .

What has all this talk of evolution got to do with germs and viruses? Viruses are the most primitive life forms known. By themselves they are inert and apparently lifeless, requiring combination with components within living cells before exhibiting lifelike characteristics. It is conjectured whether at one time they were part of the evolution of cells or whether they are unwanted remnants of the process. Viruses are of different sizes, the largest known being very

[1] Voltaire.

much smaller than the smallest bacteria (germs), which are in fact simple cells. Some bacteria are aerobic (require oxygen) and some are anaerobic, depending on whether oxygen is available to them or not, being capable of change according to the state of their immediate environment.

All living things on Earth are interdependent on other living things, the entire scenario being in a rather fine balance. The upsetting of this balance even just a little may result in the extinction of some life forms and drastic changes in others struggling to survive. We are now getting closer to the point, which is: what part of the scheme of things do germs and viruses play?

All forms of life are capable, in varying degrees, of adapting to environmental changes, and germs and viruses have been doing that from time immemorial. They are part of the scenario of life, they have a role to fill and a purpose to serve as part of Nature's "Grand Design".

When Anton van Leeuwenhoek (1632–1723) constructed one of the first effective optical microscopes, he was astounded at the complexity of miniature life forms that inhabited the world unseen to the naked eye. In a drop of clear water were myriads of tiny microbes of different kinds moving about. Similar microbes are everywhere— in the air, the soil, the water and within living tissue. Van Leeuwenhoek said: "I have had several gentlewomen in my house who are keen on seeing the little eels in vinegar [nematodes], but some of them were so disgusted at the spectacle that they vowed they would never use vinegar again. But what if one should tell such people in future that there are more animals living in the scum on the teeth in a man's mouth, than there are men in the whole kingdom?"

Thus since before the higher forms of life began to appear, the world has been teeming with bacteria (germs), which micro-organisms form the basis of all other forms of life. They manufacture soil out of rock, destroy unhealthy tissues of plants and animals, break down dead tissues of plants and animals to be used again, and actually form an essential part of the body and body functions of all animals. In this latter regard the behavior of the various forms of bacteria normal in the body is dependent on the environment within the body (which should be healthy but very often in humans is not), and it is only when the *milieu interieur* becomes deteriorated that many normal bacteria change from a benign form to a pathological form, again as a natural consequence. In Nature it is the survival of the species that counts, and individuals are expendable for the survival of the majority. The weak or sickly in the wild are not tolerated to handicap the group, and one way or another are soon eliminated by predators appointed for the purpose. C'est la vie. So when a person allows a pathological condition of body chemistry to develop within them they should realize that what follows is not a perversity of fate or an unlucky encounter with germs of a criminal nature, but merely another step in a natural sequence of events.

The scientist who in the 19th Century made the greatest contribution to the science of microbiology was Antoine Bechamp[2] (1816-1908), many of whose discoveries, all recorded in the annals of the French Academy of Science,

---

[2] Professor Pierre Jaques Antoine Bechamp, Chevalier of the Legion of Honour; Commander of the Rose of Brazil; Officer of Public Instruction; Master of Pharmacy; Doctor of Science; Doctor of Medicine; Professor of Medical Chemistry and Pharmacy, Faculty of Medicine, Montpellier; Fellow and Professor of Physics and of Toxicology Higher School of Pharmacy, Strasbourg; Professor Chemistry, Strasbourg; Member of the Imperial Academy of Medicine of France and the Society of Pharmacy of Paris; Member of the Agricultural Society of Mulhouse for the discovery of manufacturing process of aniline; Silver Medallist of the Committee of Historic works and of Learned Societies, for discoveries in wine production; Professor of Biological Chemistry and Dean of the Faculty of Medicine of Lille.

[3] *Bechamp or Pasteur? A Lost Chapter in the History of Biology* (1923) by E. Douglas Hume (founded on a manuscript by Montague R. Leverson, MD (Baltimore) MA Ph.D.

have erroneously been credited to Louis Pasteur[3] (1822–1895).

There was no love lost between the two French scientists, whose personalities were entirely different, and the record shows that although Pasteur plagiarised much of Bechamp's work, his popularity survived largely because of the favor he curried from Napoleon III and the High Church. On the other hand, Bechamp was immersed entirely in his work, seeking neither favor or fortune, and although devout in his religious faith he was held in disfavor by the Bishops of the Church, who could not comprehend the unconventional manner in which he expressed his faith.

Before Bechamp's time the theory of the cell being the basic unit of life was well established, but Bechamp's investigations showed that the cell itself was made up of smaller living entities capable of intelligent behavior and self-reproduction. He referred to these as 'molecular granulations' and gave them the name of microzymas, which he said were the real basic units of life.

Bechamp described how in certain conditions microzymas could develop into bacteria within a cell and could, if the right conditions persisted, become pathological, so that infection could develop in the body without the acquisition of the germ from an outside source. These observations supported the belief of Professor Claude Bernard (1813–78), who contended that no matter where germs came from they presented a danger only if the body was in a run-down state due to a disturbed *milieu interieur*.

Because other researchers without Bechamp's finesse had not observed the changes in form capable by various microbes, it was believed in orthodox circles that each form of the same microbe, at the time it was observed, was an entirely different microbe in its own right which remained always the same. Thus as the 19th Century came to a close, two schools of thought existed: pleomorphism as propounded by Bechamp and Ernst Almquist (1852–1946) of Sweden, and monomorphism as propounded by Pasteur and Robert Koch[4] (1843-1910) of Germany. About this time Germany became predominant in world medical research, and because the germ theory of disease had become firmly entrenched in the minds of orthodox doctors, the research into microbiology became focussed more on medical problems than on the general study of biology.

Nevertheless, evidence supporting the concept of pleomorphism kept appearing.[5] In 1907 Doctors A. Neisser and Rudolph Massine described the mutation-like phenomena in a strain of B coli, and in 1914 Philip Eisenberg published a series of papers on bacterial variability. A similar study was published in 1918 by bacteriologist Karl Baerthlein, which later received high praise from Dr Phillip Hadley, University of Pittsburg, in his paper "Microbic Disassociation" (Journal of Infectious Diseases, Vol. 40, 1927).

In 1898, Guenther Enderlein (1872-1968) graduated with honors in natural sciences, physics and zoology from Leipzig University, and in 1914 he became a bacteriologist and serologist at the German military hospital at Stettin. Enderlein had studied the findings of Antoine Bechamp and had further studied under Rudolph Leuckart, the zoologist who initiated the modern science of parasitology, and also under Otto Schmidt, the doctor who in 1901 reported the discovery of parasites in the blood of cancer patients. (Schmidt was not the first to discover cancer parasites. As early as 1890 Scottish pathologist William Russell reported on widely variegated microbes present in

---

[4] Robert Koch (*see* footnote p. 72) had noted but never investigated the pleomorphic forms of the typhoid bacillus.

[5] In the chapter which follows it is described how in the study of the disease beriberi, ten different researchers reported they had discovered the germ that caused the disease. Each germ was different and none of them turned out to be the cause at all, but what is indicated is the probability that at least some of the microbes isolated from beriberi patients represented different stages of pleomorphism.

all cancer tissue, which microbes were referred to as "Russell bodies".)

It was in 1916 while studying typhus that Dr Enderlein observed microscopic living entities in blood samples which he called protits, which could move, unite with other micro-organisms and disappear. Later on, using dark field microscopy, he observed that these micro-organisms could change in form through a cycle of countless variations, and he also described how different types of protein-based micro-organisms flourished in blood cells and plasma of all animals, representing an essential part of the normal life process. As part of the normal life process, these micro-organisms live together within the body in a mutually beneficial relationship known as symbiosis. However, he noted that with any deterioration of the body's interior environment in which the pH of the blood becomes either acid or strongly alkaline,[6] the normally harmless microbes would begin to change and in stages evolve into forms of a pathogenic nature, just as Bechamp had said. Enderlein recorded these observations in his book *Bakterien Cyclogenic (The Life Cycle of Bacteria)*, published in 1925 (translated from the German by Dr Phillip Hadley), at which time he became a member of the Microbiological Society of Vienna of which he was later to become president.

[6] Cholera is a disease characterized by the onset of diarrhoea and occurs in different degrees from mild to fatal; the etiology of the mild forms is uncertain in the presence of varying kinds of bacilli (germs) but Asiatic or true cholera is transmitted by a bacillus called *Vibrio cholera*, a member of a large group of gram-negative, comma-shaped bacteria that are morphologically indistinguishable from one another. Some of these bacteria appear normally and symbiotically in the body and are often found associated with mild diarrhoea. However, true cholera can be transmitted by a germ different to *Vibrio cholera* called *El Tor vibrio* which, unlike *Vibrio cholera*, can be found in the absence of disease as well. Another fact about the cholera germ which further supports Dr Enderlein's thesis is that it thrives best in a strongly alkaline milieu.

Dr Enderlein's sixty years of research using more refined equipment achieved discoveries which precisely duplicated those of Bechamp and confirmed Bechamp's views. Enderlein found that:

1 The cell does not represent the primary living unit of the body. Instead the primary units were tiny biological units which he called protits which live within the cells.
2 The blood is not sterile, but contains micro-organisms capable of causing mischief given the proper milieu.
3 Certain micro-organisms undergo an exact, scientifically verifiable growth cycle.

Presently Dr Enderlein's findings continue to be confirmed by Dr Erik Enby of Gothenburg, Sweden, where he practises biological medicine and is assistant physician at the Vasa Hospital. Dr Enby's observations of micro-organisms are done using interference contrasting microscopy.

Shortly after *Bakterien Cyclogenic* was published, American researchers F. Loenis and N.R. Smith collaborated to write *Studies of the Life Cycles of Bacteria*, which Enderlein welcomed as sufficient support to finally finish the pleomorphism vs monomorphism argument, but as always the orthodox medical establishment was not interested in anything which did not agree with the textbooks and the monomorphic dogma contained therein.

Another "medical heretic" was Dr William F. Koch, BA MA Ph.D MD,[7] of Detroit, whose life's work was the study of the biochemistry in disease. In his book *The Survival Factor in Neoplastic and Viral Diseases* (1961) he says:

"Glover showed in 1923 that the cancer virus existed in a pleomorphic form that was a bacillus in one phase and coccus in another, and virus in the third phase. He also showed it could exist in a fungus or mycelium phase. The latter form has been identified lately by Irene Diller and some others,

[7] *See* Chapter 12.

and the whole chain of forms was independently proved by von Brehmer in the last few decades as well. The work was thoroughly repeated and proved by my friend Jacob Engel and George Clark, at the US PHS Laboratories but, for reasons we will not discuss, they were not allowed to publish their findings."

In 1933, Dr Wilhelm von Brehmer stated his belief in the theory that cancer was a constitutional disease related to diet and lifestyle, and in his book *Sipohonospora Polymorpha von Brehmer* he identified this blood parasite (S.p.), a bacterial form of the fungi *Mucor racemosus*, as a carcinogenic agent present in cancerous growth. His research showed that excessive alkalinity of the blood permitted lower forms of mucor to develop into pathogenic rods. (When S.p. was again discovered by Dr Virginia Livingstone Wheeler of San Diego she called it "Progenitor Cryptocides", while other doctors just called it the cancer microbe.)

Not only cancer, but all chronic pathological conditions display in the blood various pleomorphic micro-organisms which originate from within the body itself to proliferate and participate in the disease process. Dr Raymond Brown, formerly of the Sloan Kettering Institute for Cancer Research, in his book *AIDS, Cancer, and the Medical Establishment* (1986) says:

"Pleomorphic organisms are demonstrable as the silent stage of a gamut of infections that include Tuberculosis, Syphilis, Leprosy, Rheumatic Fever, Undulant Fever, Typhoid, and Candida. They have been repeatedly found in diseases of undetermined etiology: Arthritis, Cancer, Multiple Sclerosis, Sarcoid Collagen Disease, Whipple's Disease, Crohn's Disease, and Kaposi's Sarcoma."

Additional up-to-date information on pleomorphism is revealed in the 1981 book *Symbiosis in Cell Evolution* by Dr Lynn Margulis of Boston University:

"A very few eukaryotes[8] and protoctists, and a few
fungi, are tolerant to anaerobic conditions, but
under such conditions the mitochondria shrink
(sometimes until they are invisible) and become
non-functional. This differentiation is reversible;
the organisms retain the capacity to re-differentiate
the mitochondria."

to anaerobic conditions, but under such conditions the
mitochondria shrink (sometimes until they are invisible)
and become non-functional. This differentiation is
reversible; the organisms retain the capacity to re-
differentiate the mitochondria."

It was the constant observations of differently
described microbes in the blood and tissues of cancer
patients that eventually prompted the US National Institute
of Health to launch a full-scale investigation as to whether
cancer was virus caused, which investigation in the 1970s
(President Nixon's War Against Cancer) showed that the
so-called cancer virus was resultant to the disturbed body
chemistry which precedes cancer and not the cause of it,
a fact stated over the last hundred years by many
distinguished cancer researchers.

That germs from outside the body can cause disease
in susceptible people is not disputed. There are many
instances of epidemics so caused, such as the cholera
epidemic of 1854 in Lambeth, London, when water
supplied by one particular street pump became con-
taminated by a cesspool, and many people using that pump
came down with cholera, while people nearby, using a
different supply, suffered no cholera. The epidemic stopped
as soon as the pump was de-activated.

Probably the most well-known case of infection by
human contact occurred not long before that in 1847 when
there was an appalling death rate among women in
childbirth at a hospital in Vienna. The doctor in charge,

---

[8] Eukaryotes are cells which have a nucleus; prokaryotes are cells
which have no nucleus.

Ignaz Semmelweis,[9] realized that the cause of the puerperal sepsis infecting women was that many of the doctors were in the habit of attending the women immediately after having been vivisecting corpses elsewhere in the hospital and that none of them washed their hands. When Semmelweis insisted all doctors must wash their hands in chlorinated water before attending at childbirths, the death rate among mothers dropped quickly from 18% to less than 3%.

This case is particularly interesting because it demonstrates not only the cases both for and against the germ theory, but at the same time the case for pleomorphism, the changing of microbes from one form into another. A healthy body's *milieu interieur* is alkaline in nature with a pH of 7.2–7.6 (7.0 being neutral), any variation either way tending towards disease. In acidic conditions morbidity increases in proportion to acidity, and after death the acidity becomes much stronger, providing

[9] Semmelweis was not the first to realize the cause of puerperal sepsis. Dr Charles White of Manchester had come to the correct conclusion in 1773, and by 1835 Dr Robert Collins of Ireland had effectively reduced mortality among women in childbirth in his hospital in Dublin. Oliver Wendell Holmes, philosopher, poet and physician, while Professor of Anatomy at Dartmouth College, USA, also concluded that puerperal sepsis resulted from doctors proceeding direct to conducting childbirths without washing their hands after treating septic wounds elsewhere in the hospital. He had observed as well that it was not uncommon for doctors to suffer infection, sometimes fatal, after having cut themselves accidentally while performing an autopsy. Holmes wrote a heated paper on the topic in 1843, which was put down as nonsense by the so-called experts on childbed fever, and he republished the paper titled "Puerperal Fever as a Private Pestilence" in 1855, which although again rejected by the medical establishment thereafter gradually gained acceptance.

Semmelweis' ideas were never accepted in Austria during his lifetime and he died of blood poisoning from a wound in the hand in 1865.

the environment for the body to decompose. The dead tissues self-destruct in the process called autolysis under the influence of the natural enzyme, cathepsin, and the action of natural bacteria which appear automatically when the acid condition occurs. Where do these bacteria come from? Answer: they have been in the body all the time but in a different form which is harmless.

They are the bacteria *Mucor racemosus fresen* which, as stated by Dr Enderlein and Dr von Brehmer, change in form according to the state of the *milieu interieur*, from its harmless, symbiotic stage through a number of other stages (which are reversible) to become pathogenic and finally tissue destructive. In this final phase the bacteria, now resembling a fungus, is most pathogenic, and on the unwashed hands of the doctors from the dissecting room were a lethal threat to anyone susceptible to them.

But not every woman in Semmelweis' maternity section was susceptible, and even at the worst time, eighty-two out of a hundred escaped the deadly puerperal sepsis. Many hundreds of people in Lambeth died of cholera in the cholera epidemic; they were the susceptible ones—the unsusceptible ones escaped.

Maybe a better illustration of susceptibility and unsusceptibility is given by Sir Albert Howard in his book *The Role of Insects and Fungi in Agriculture*. In the livestock industry, foot and mouth disease is considered so deadly that entire herds are destroyed and burned once the disease appears in any of the animals to prevent it spreading to other farms. But Sir Albert had this to say:

"For twenty one years [1910–31] I was able to study the reaction of well-fed animals to epidemic diseases, such as rinderpest, foot-and-mouth disease, septicemia and so forth, which frequently devastated the countryside. None of my animals were segregated, none were inoculated; they frequently came in contact with diseased stock. No case of infectious disease occurred. The reward of well-nourished protoplasm was a very high degree of

disease resistance; which might even be described
as immunity."

In his book *Soil, Grass and Cancer* (Crosby Lockwood,
London, 1959), French author Andre Voisin, biochemist
and agriculturist, demonstrated how health and disease are
related to the soil via the nutritional quality of the crops
produced thereon. In regard to foot and mouth disease in
cattle, Voisin quoted German and French data showing
the disease hardly ever occurred in granite and sandy
regions, but that sometimes in soils high in lime it affected
up to eighty per cent of animals. The susceptibility to the
disease Voisin ascribed to copper deficiency, which
prevented the animals producing enough catalase, the
predominant protective enzyme of the immune system.

Similar examples of lowered catalase in both humans
and animals that permitted otherwise harmless germs to
act pathogenically to produce different disease symptoms
were given, and as the title of the book indicates, the
importance of trace minerals in the prevention of cancer
was emphasized.

In regard to tuberculosis Voisin said:

> "The lungs of each one of us are inhabited by
> millions of tuberculosis bacilli, which we manage
> to accommodate quite well. They live there very
> peacefully without delivering frenzied attacks
> against our cells. Why then, do they suddenly thrust
> themselves upon one of our organs (most often the
> lungs) and make us tuberculosis sufferers?"

Voisin then went on to demonstrate how defective
nutrition is the underlying problem, the milk from
tuberculous cows having no bearing on the matter because
the human victim's bacillus is already present, with or
without the milk. As for the tuberculous cows, they do
not have to be destroyed; like their human counterparts
all they need is better pastures and conditions.

That healthy humans are every bit as disease resistant
as healthy farm animals is borne out by an extract from

the book *Immune for Life* by Arnold Fox, MD, of Los
Angeles, former Assistant Professor of Medicine, University
of California, Irvine:

> "Many years ago, as a resident in Internal Medicine
> at Los Angeles County Hospital, I was in charge
> of the adult infectious-disease ward. For ten to
> fifteen hours a day, I was exposed to just about
> every infectious illness you can imagine. These
> patients had tuberculosis, meningitis, the very
> deadly septicemia and other dangerous diseases.
> They coughed and sneezed on me; I got their blood,
> sweat and even feces on my hands. But I didn't
> 'catch' any of their diseases. My 'doctor within' kept
> me in perfect health.
>
> Some time later I was transferred from the
> infectious-disease ward and into surgery. Months
> later I came down with meningitis, a potentially
> deadly infection of the covering of the brain. I hadn't
> been near anyone with meningitis who could have
> 'given' me the disease. What happened was that I
> was working double shifts, going to every class and
> lecture offered, and moonlighting as well. I had
> run my immune system down to the ground."

The experience of Dr Fox is not unique, being
common to all doctors, nurses and other hospital staff all
around the world, and the great wonder of medicine is
that Pasteur's germ theory of disease holds on in peoples'
minds the way it does.

That a healthy body can resist infection even in
unhygienic circumstances seems to surprise a lot of people,
the author's wife included. Recently I was engaged in
unloading some old planks from my truck, and I ripped
my right index finger to the bone just above the knuckle
on a rusty nail. As the blood spurted out I could see the
cut needed stitching, but I figured I would finish unloading
the truck if I could stem the bleeding. In the truck was
some old rag I had tied around some garden stakes so I

tore off a strip, bandaged the wound and finished unloading. Back at the house my wife insisted I should go to the local hospital to have the wound sterilised, stitched and so forth, to escape the "deadly" tetanus[10] germ, but as by this time the bleeding had stopped completely, I simply rebandaged the wound over the dried blood and dirt without so much as washing it, and put my trust in Nature. I recalled that as a boy my frequent wounds sometimes festered and took ages to heal but now over fifty years later I figured I was healthier and things would be different. The wound would of course have been better stitched because my hand movements would not permit it to close properly, but nevertheless it healed completely in a bit over a week but left an ugly scar which made me regret not having it stitched. However, I was surprised that as a few more weeks went

---

[10] The reason why people with good blood need have no fear of tetanus is made clear in a statement taken from Dr Otto Warburg's lecture "The Prime Cause and Prevention of Cancer" given at the meeting of Nobel Laureates at Landau, Germany, on 30 June 1966 (*see* Chapter 12):

"If it is true that the replacement of oxygen-respiration by fermentation is the prime cause of cancer, then all cancer cells without exception must ferment, and no normal growing cell ought to exist that ferments in the body.

An especially simple and convincing experiment performed by the Americans Malmgren and Flanegan confirms that view. *If one injects tetanus spores, which can germinate only at very low oxygen pressures, into the blood of healthy mice, the mice do not sicken with tetanus, because the spores find no place in the normal body where the oxygen pressure is sufficiently low* . . . However, if one injects tetanus spores into the blood of tumor-bearing mice, the mice sicken with tetanus, because the oxygen pressure in the tumors can be so low that the spores can germinate. These experiments demonstrate in a unique way the anaerobiosis of cancer cells and the non-anaerobioses of normal cells."

by the raised scar diminished so that now only the faintest suggestion of a scar remains.

The reason my hand did not become infected was that I am not susceptible to infection, which is why I never "catch" colds or flu either.

Thus it becomes very clear that the real cause of infectious diseases is whatever it is that renders a person susceptible. And we know what that something is: it is the absence of homeostasis in the body brought about by a disturbed *milieu interieur*.

"The body is the temple of the soul", so it is said, and germs are natural inhabitants of it, some of which assist in the day to day running of the temple and some which, when the temple begins to decay, perform to more quickly complete its destruction.

As Robert Ingersoll said: "In Nature there are neither rewards or punishments. There are consequences."

Addendum to Germs and Viruses

If I could live my life over again, I would devote it to proving that germs seek their natural habitat, diseased tissue, rather than being the cause of the diseased tissue.
                    Rudolph Virchow (1821–1902)

The long-standing confusion about germs can be understood when it is considered that, even within the restrictions limiting the powers of visual light microscopes (as compared to the electron microscope), there are worlds within worlds, depending on which range of magnification is being explored and whether the design of the microscope permits the study of living tissue (blood and cells) or only that which is dead.

Dr Abraham Baron, B.Sc MSc Ph.D, Professor of bacteriology, biochemistry and physiology at Long Island University 1935–1941, wrote the book *Man Against Germs* (1958, Robert Hale, London) in which he describes "monomorphically" the different microbes and the diseases associated with them. Then right at the end in the final chapter on Q Fever, to Dr Baron's puzzlement, pleomorphism enters the scene:

> "These germs, a new and unusual species of Rickettsia, are extraordinary; they are remarkably adaptable and incredibly vigorous. They can assume any size and any shape, sub-dividing into almost invisible granules as small as the smallest of the viruses, or growing out into large coarse filaments, but in any form their virulence remains undiminished. They can infect any species of animal, animal to man, or man to man. The full account of their potentialities *still escapes the formulae of science and medicine. Q Fever is more than just a disease; it is the key to a law of Nature.*" (author's italics)

Then in his final paragraphs, Professor Baron (without knowing it) described Antoine Bechamp's microzymas, which but for the dogmatism of Pasteur and Koch he would have learned about at medical school instead of at the end of his career:

> "Within the protoplasm of our living cells, there is a miscellany of small strange particles that vaguely resemble bits of string, or tiny spheres, or miniature corkscrews. And ever since the microscope was discovered, many generations of scientists have peered and poured over them and disputed their significance. Some claim that these particles in the human protoplasm are extremely important, possessing certain vital (but unspecified) functions, while others believe they are trivial with trivial functions. And still others insist that these particles have no function at all, that they are shadowy "nothings" that exist only in the overwrought imaginings of over-enthusiastic scientists, or as imperfections in their microscopes, their straining

eyes or their laboratory technique. Although the embattled scientists agree neither on the status or the functions of these protoplasmic particles, they are compelled to agree at the least on a *casus belli*, even if only to deny that it exists. The most bitter opponents of their existence must call these strange particles something, and so some of them have been named—*centrioles, mitochondria, nucleoli, plastids, vacuoles, inclusions, Golgi network, granules, globules, filaments, fibers, fibrilles, and "ad infinitum"*.

There are other scientists who study human protoplasm in quite another manner and are completely uninterested in the particles within the human living cells. From their researches on immunity to disease, they have deduced that certain germs (the viruses of poliomyelitis, for example) first infect and cause disease and thereafter never leave the human body. Then the germs no longer cause disease, but they remain alive though inert for a human lifetime.

There is still another school of scientists who probe into the disputed interior of living human cells. They have discovered that they can extract germs from healthy uninfected, undiseased human cells. The germs they extract are alive and will grow on human tissue, but never cause disease. The scientists are convinced that there are always living germs buried deeply within human protoplasm."

And so, more puzzled at the end of his long career than he was as a student, but ever so close to the answer he was seeking, Professor Baron concludes his book:

"If we have correctly interpreted Nature's law, then all our disease germs will change from antagonism to co-existence, and turn from dangerous bits of alien life into inconspicuous particles within our living cells. Perhaps far ahead in the future in a

disease-free world, the descendants of germs and
men will live together harmoniously in a mingling
of protoplasm—a perfect symbiosis of men and
germs.''

I have included Professor Baron's remarks for two very
important reasons. Without realizing it, the professor has
illustrated clearly the fundamental errors in thinking that
have prevented any worthwhile progress in medicine for
over one hundred years:

1 The unswerving belief in the monomorphic nature of
germs despite all the evidence they are polymorphic, a
phenomenon witnessed and described by Professor Baron
himself.
2 The belief that germs and viruses are "dangerous bits
of alien life" out to harm us.

The professor has indeed correctly interpreted Nature's
laws insofar as Nature is desirous that germs and men
should co-exist harmoniously, but he fails to realize that
to achieve this state of "perfect symbiosis" we do not have
to look far ahead into the future at all, because it is available
to us right now and always has been. Whether germs behave
like dangerous bits of alien life or like inconspicuous
particles is entirely up to us and how we choose to look
after our *milieu interieur.*

And in case you think that antibiotics and vaccines
offer a way to cheat the system, I suggest that would be
as dangerous an error as ever medical science has devised.
Nature cannot be fooled, and her justice is
uncompromising.

CHAPTER 6

Human Errors and Human Ills

*If a little knowledge is dangerous, where is the
man who has so much as to be out of danger?*
Thomas Huxley (1825–95)

When assessing any situation it should always be
remembered that very often things are not always as they
may at first seem. "There are more things than meet the
eye." To err is human, and conclusions hastily arrived at
often turn out to be wrong. The reason that the practice
of medicine fails to accomplish its purpose—the
elimination of human disease—is that its concepts are
based, almost entirely, on false conclusions.

Take the case of an old lady who falls over one day
and breaks a hip bone. So? She fell over and broke her
hip, isn't that obvious? But hold on a minute—the old
lady has osteoporosis, her bones are brittle and weak, so
weak in fact that the bone snapped under her weight and
that's why she fell over. That's not so obvious. In any case,
the bone was weak because it lacked calcium, so she is
advised to drink lots of milk and take calcium tablets to
strengthen her bones. That seems to make sense, but again,
hold on a minute. The lady's diet already has as much
calcium in it as anyone else's, so could there be another
reason her bones are lacking in it? Yes, there is—the lady's
lifelong diet was high in protein, which she had always
been told was a good thing, but nobody told her that protein

was acid forming in the body and in the amounts commonly consumed so much acid is formed that the body is forced to "borrow" calcium from the bones in order to neutralize it. That's why heavy protein-eaters get osteoporosis as they age, and why most vegetarians do not. Nobody told her either that the calcium from calcium tables does not strengthen the bones and that a lot of it, together with the fat in the milk, only helps to worsen her atherosclerosis which again due to her diet she would undoubtedly have.

It is commonly believed that heredity is a major factor in degenerative diseases such as heart disease, cancer, diabetes, etc. That it is a major factor seems obvious when you can easily observe how these diseases run in families. But again, things are not always as they seem. Just as different countries have different traditional foods, so too are family eating habits, acquired in childhood, passed on within families from generation to generation, and it is mainly by way of these passed on habits that a predisposition to a certain disease continues to run in families, not because of inherited characteristics. In Japan the incidence of stomach cancer is much higher than in the US, not because Japanese are more genetically prone to it than are Americans but because of their traditional highly salted diet. And in the US, colon (bowel) cancer and heart disease are much more common than in Japan, not because Americans are genetically prone to these diseases, but because of their traditional high-protein, high-fat diet. Therefore, a young Japanese who migrates to the US and adopts the American diet will have a very high chance of getting colon cancer and heart disease but a very low chance of getting stomach cancer, regardless of how many of his forebears back in Japan have died of stomach cancer.

But as the Japanese become wealthier and consume more and more meat in their diet, so their death rates from heart disease and colon cancer are gradually increasing.

In disease research there are always red herrings to lead us to wrong conclusions. Take lung cancer for instance. What causes lung cancer? Smoking? Sure, smokers are more prone to lung cancer—or any cancer—than non-smokers, but how is it that the Japanese, who are heavier smokers than Europeans and Americans, have a much lower incidence of lung cancer? Answer: because the traditional Japanese diet is very low in fat and cholesterol, and this answer was proved many years ago in a Chicago study of 876 smokers which showed that smokers with cholesterol levels over 7.1 mmol/l (275 m/%) had a lung cancer rate seven times higher than smokers with levels below 5.8 (225 m/%), and for those smokers with cholesterol levels below 3.9 (150) the lung cancer rate was zero. Same thing with skin cancer. The rate of skin cancer has increased over the years, not because the sun has become hotter, but because of a higher consumption of fat, protein and cholesterol. It is the increased toxemia and reduced blood circulation to the tissues resultant to these dietary errors that render the tissue cells unhealthy and pre-cancerous, whereupon some form of local irritation or injury may trigger them to become cancerous. In the case of lung cancer and skin cancer it is the smoke and sunshine, respectively, that provide the trigger action.

Diabetes is another example of jumping to false conclusions. When in 1889 it was demonstrated in medical experiments that dogs with their pancreas removed immediately displayed the symptoms of diabetes, and when in 1921 it was discovered that the hormone insulin injected into such dogs removed the symptoms, it became clear to the researchers that diabetes was a disease caused by a defective pancreas not producing enough insulin. Since then the standard treatment for diabetes has been the injection of insulin by hypodermic needle. Simple. In this way diabetics can lead fairly normal lives but, although their lives are extended, diabetics are still very prone to blindness and fatal circulatory disorders. If insulin is not the answer to diabetes but only a crutch to keep diabetics going, then what is the answer?

The answer has been known for over one hundred years and is easy to understand once all the factors are taken into account. The elevated blood sugar which is the main indicator of diabetes shows that the sugar which the body desperately needs is there in plenty but something is preventing the body using it. Medical training tells doctors that the problem is lack of insulin from a defective pancreas, despite the fact it has long been known that most diabetics produce normal or even greater amounts of insulin. Obviously the answer to the problem lies somewhere else.

Over one hundred years ago, Louis Kuhne of Germany and other perceptive doctors like Charles de Lacy Evans and Emmet Densmore of England and Edward Dewey of the USA[1] were successfully "curing" diabetics of their problem by dietary means, it being obvious to them that diabetes was mainly a dietary problem. It was no coincidence that with the disappearance of the patients' diabetic symptoms so too did other symptoms of disease disappear. Dr Albert Schweitzer was a diabetic and his wife had tuberculosis. In 1928 both were "cured" of their diseases by Dr Max Gerson using the diet which he had found so effective in curing lupus and cancer. (*See The Health Revolution* and *Improving on Pritikin* by Ross Horne.)

In the 1920s it was discovered that the main factor in preventing the metabolism of blood sugar in the presence of normal insulin was too much fat in the blood, and in 1936 Dr I.M. Rabinowitch of Canada presented 1000 case studies demonstrating this to the Diabetic Association in Boston, whose only action was to ignore them. Other studies showed that fit young athletes could be made diabetic in only two days on a diet loaded with fat and protein and just as quickly normalized when the excess fat and protein were eliminated. Stress and inactivity were exacerbating factors. Only when Nathan Pritikin dug out this information in the 1960s was it put to good use, when Pritikin later demonstrated that eighty per cent of long-term diabetics put on a low-fat diet could be taken off their

---

[1] Louis Kuhne, author of *The New Science of Healing*; Charles de Lacy Evans, author of *How to Prolong Life*; Emmet Densmore, author of *How Nature Cures*; Edward Dewey, author of *The True Science of Living*.

medication entirely in less than four weeks. Since then, in Australia, tests have demonstrated that diabetic, city-dwelling Aboriginals, when relocated in their tribal lands and resuming their native diet, quickly become completely free of diabetes.

In 1852 Dr A. Coccius published data on the association of "agglutinated" blood with human disease, and in the 1940s Dr Melvin Knisely of the University of Chicago published a series of papers describing the association of "sludged" blood with over fifty common degenerative diseases. Other doctors like Meyer Friedman of San Francisco and Leopold Dintenfas of Sydney have over the last thirty years published similar findings showing "high viscosity" blood to be involved with degenerative diseases such as heart disease, diabetes, cancer, hypertension, rheumatoid arthritis, asthma, glaucoma and multiple sclerosis. Routine everyday blood tests show that high sedimentation rates (ESR) and high platelet adhesion index (PAI), which reflect high blood viscosity, accompany chronic diseases. Medical journals have published information describing how heart patients maintained for years on digitalis to enhance their blood flow suffer only one tenth the cancer incidence of comparable patients not on digitalis. Observe how patients too ill to eat for a few days rapidly improve, only to deteriorate when their appetite for a "good dinner" returns.

Toxemia, blood sludge, high blood viscosity—if doctors are aware of it at all, their medical training leads them to believe the condition is resultant of the "disease", when in fact it is the other way around—it *is* the disease. How impure, sludged blood results in the individual symptoms called arthritis, hypertension and so on I have described in detail in my book *The Health Revolution*, and the proof that the principles of natural health work is contained in the sheaves of letters sent me by grateful people now free of their problems.

By now the reader may suspect that all medical theory is based on false conclusions drawn without complete appraisal of the available evidence, and it is the author's aim to demonstrate this is the case, not only in regard to degenerative and metabolic diseases but also in regard to so-called infectious diseases, including AIDS. The puzzlement of medical scientists struggling today to "defeat" AIDS, hepatitis, leukemia and so on is the same puzzlement that confounded the medical scientists a hundred years ago in their attempts to solve the problem of beriberi, and the puzzlement will continue as long as they continue to repeat the same 100-year-old mistake . . .

Beriberi is a disease characterized by weakness, nervous disorders, a swollen liver, weight loss, paralysis and impaired heart action. Until well into the 20th Century beriberi caused untold loss of life mainly in Asia and the East Indies, where rice forms the basis of the traditional diet. In 1878 Pasteur had announced his germ theory of disease, and so convincingly did he present it that it quickly found acceptance in the French Academy of Science and in a short time became part of established medical dogma around the world. From this time on, medical research became almost entirely directed into identifying which germ caused which disease so that a vaccine could be manufactured to defeat the germ and cure the disease. It was at this very time the Dutch government was concerned about the enormous death toll from beriberi in their colonies, and the Japanese navy was likewise concerned about the heavy losses of seamen from the same cause, and great efforts were being made to identify the germ responsible. However, in Java in 1887 it was discovered by a young physician, Christiaan Eijkman, that beriberi was not caused by a germ at all but by a diet deficiency correctable by eating unpolished rice instead of polished rice, and in Japan at the same time a naval physician, Kanehiro Takaki, made the same discovery. The problem of beriberi was solved, except for one thing—nobody took any notice because the medical establishment decreed a germ was responsible and a germ must be found.

Unfortunately for Eijkman (and a lot of other people), his superior, Professor Pekalharing, had already in 1887 discovered a germ he claimed caused beriberi, which he called the "bacillus beriberi"; there were other similar claims as well. To quote researcher James Le Fanu: "Glockner identified an amoeba, Thaardo a haematozoan, Pereira a spherical micro-organism, Durham a looped streptococcus, Taylor a spirillum, Winkler a staphylococcus, and Dangerfield an aerobic micrococcus." In addition, in 1901 Van de Scheer reported a virus, and in 1903 Maurex discovered a "fungus". Each of these researchers was convinced the germ they had found was the cause of beriberi, and every one of them was mistaken.

It was Casimer Funk in 1911 who extracted the mysterious factor from rice bran that prevented beriberi, but for many more years the death toll continued in Asia and the Philippines and as late as 1925, thirty-eight years after Kanehiro Takaki's discovery, beriberi was still causing 15,000 deaths per year in Japan. The concept of deficiency diseases was eventually accepted in medical circles in about 1929, and it was in 1934 that chemist R.R. Williams of the USA isolated Funk's X factor from rice bran and called it thiamine, or vitamin B_1.

The same story can be told about scurvy, the disease that destroyed thousands of seafarers until authorities realized that Captain Cook was right in feeding his men lime juice and green vegetables. And the same story is that of the disease rickets, shown by French physician Armand Trousseau to be preventable by taking fish liver oil. For many years after these discoveries it was still thought in medical circles that the diseases were attributable to germs.

Some diseases of dietary origin are caused by an effect similar to outright poisoning. Gluten in wheat severely affects some people and no doubt in some degree is harmful to everybody, but the chemical make up of corn is worse. Pellagra is a disease common among people whose diet is based heavily on corn and corn products, and is characterized by soreness of the mouth and tongue, inflammation of the digestive tract, diarrhea, mental disturbances and discoloration of the skin. As far back as 1735 it was known in Europe that pellagra resulted from a diet mainly of corn, and yet in 1914 the death rate from pellagra among the poverty-stricken sharecroppers in south-eastern USA, who were dependent on corn for food, reached 1000 per month with the medical profession continuing to insist the disease was caused by germs. It was only in 1916 when Dr Joseph Goldberger of the US Public Health Service injected himself with a solution made from the scabs of pellagra patients, with no subsequent ill effects, that the germ theory was finally ruled out— that is, for pellagra. It has been shown since then that corn is not only deficient in many nutritional aspects, but at the same time contains an unidentified substance toxic in the body.

The germ theory is a deficient theory because it only seems to work part of the time while for most of the time it doesn't hold at all, whether either germs or viruses are the objects of suspicion. There are many different viruses associated with the common cold,[2] but not everyone exposed to them gets a cold. There is a germ associated with tuberculosis, but few people exposed to it get tuberculosis. There are a number of different bacteria associated with cholera,[3] but not everybody exposed to them gets cholera. There are viruses associated with hepatitis, germs and viruses associated with venereal diseases, and so on, but not everyone contacting these germs and viruses gets the disease they are supposed to. Some do, some don't.

When the germ theory was first promulgated, Robert Koch (1843–1910),[4] the famous bacteriologist of the 19th

[2] Tests in which cold viruses have been inserted directly into the nasal passages of volunteer subjects showed that colds could be passed from one person to another, depending on the fitness of the recipient. In one test with twelve volunteers, $33\frac{1}{3}$ per cent developed colds, in another with thirty-six subjects, 42 per cent developed colds, and in a group of thirty-six students, only 2.8 per cent developed colds.

[3] Susceptibility to cholera (see Chapter 5) varies widely and is markedly influenced by predisposing factors such as low gastric acidity, pre-existing gastro-intestinal disorders and alcoholism.

[4] Robert Koch discovered the germ associated with anthrax in cattle, and the germs held responsible for tuberculosis and cholera in humans.

Century, laid down a set of rules called Koch's Postulates which had to be met in order to prove a certain germ caused a certain disease. The postulates were:

1 The microbe (germ) must be found in all cases of disease, but not in healthy subjects.
2 It must be isolated from the patient and grown in culture.
3 It must be introduced to a new host and in that host produce the original disease.
4 It must be found present in the host so infected.

But when these rules were rigidly applied it was apparent that the germ theory was inconsistent, as we have seen, so the third postulate was changed to saying the germ had to produce the original disease in a *susceptible* new host.

With the addition of the single word "susceptible" the entire concept of the germ theory is changed. The accent is taken away from the germ and placed on the word susceptibility, not only susceptibility of the second host but also that of the first host—in other words, for a germ to cause a disease in anybody, at any time, it can only do so if the person is susceptible. Thus Koch agreed with his friend Pasteur who, before he died, admitted that "Bernard was right, the germ is nothing, the milieu is everything."

So having come to agreement that germs and viruses pose a threat only to susceptible subjects, it remains only to clarify what susceptible means. Susceptibility is a condition of lowered health and vitality which exists when the homeostasis of the body becomes disharmonised due to undesirable changes in the *milieu interieur*. As the *milieu interieur* changes rapidly for better or worse according to what is eaten and many other factors, so susceptibility may vary or be chronic, which explains why some sick people go 'in and out of remission' and why some remain chronic.

From all of the past errors in medical thinking, what good, if any, has eventuated? Not much. The medical establishment is not even aware it may be on the wrong track, and that is the biggest error of all. Medical thinking is still disease/cure oriented instead of lifestyle/health oriented. Medical researchers, bankrupt of results, still deliver promises only: "imminent breakthroughs", "exciting new prospects", "in less than ten years", etc, while others, weary of being confused by viruses, now seek to track down the "defective genes" that "cause the immune system to turn against itself". And so on. The show goes on, it is a flop, and the tickets are expensive.

Whereas the purpose of this chapter has been to highlight some of the gross errors in thinking upon which current medical practice is still based, the reason for doing this is to instil in the minds of everyone the deepest suspicion of all forms of medical treatment and all statements and claims issued from the entrenched medical establishment, the members of which, by and large, are as deluded by their own mumbo jumbo as those they feed it to in good faith.

The worst part of the tragedy is not that people die long before their appointed potential span is up, but that so many suffer so much mental and physical distress before they do so. Life is not meant to be like that, but it will always be so while we wallow in ignorance.

The reader will no doubt have found some of the foregoing disclosures surprising, even hard to believe, but others equally surprising are yet to follow, which all put together prove one thing at least: which is, in the words of Dr William Roe of New Zealand from his book *Science in Medical Practise* (1984):

> "No more than a superficial acquaintance with anthropology, ethnology, or history is required for it to become apparent that the need to indulge in fantasy is deeply ingrained in man. Indeed it seems the most distinctive (and perhaps the most dangerous) characteristic of that species of the genus Homo we conceitedly label Sapiens is not his wisdom but his reluctance to admit ignorance. Rather than do so, he is prone to prosit an hypothesis and, all too frequently in the absence

of supporting evidence, comes to believe it. Thus
are myths created."

The myth of germs and viruses as primary disease
agents has existed now for over 100 years. Viruses now take
the spotlight. Billions of dollars have been spent trying
to annihilate them before they annihilate us! The common
cold, herpes, hepatitis, glandular fever, AIDS—all defy
medical science. The hepatitis C virus is the latest one to
gain the distinction of "deadly". Who is at risk from
"deadly" hepatitis C? Why, none other than intravenous
drug users, people who have had blood transfusions, renal
dialysis patients and—wait for it—male homosexuals!
These are the sort of people who get AIDS: their immune
systems are low, they are susceptible people.

When will the penny drop? The reason modern
medicine cannot "cure" viral diseases is that they are not
caused by viruses. The viruses are there all right but, in
the words of Dr Richard Ablin (*see* Chapter 7), "they may
turn out to be passengers on an already sinking ship".

The same confusion that confounded medical research
in the past still exists today about viruses and their
association with hepatitis, herpes, the common cold and
various other symptoms contained in the AIDS problem.
These so-called agents of disease are, like the germs of
cholera, tuberculosis and beriberi, certainly to be found
in sick people but they are no more the direct cause of
the disease than flies are the cause of garbage. So is explained
how various microbes and viruses are often detectable living
acquiescently in the blood of healthy people, even newborn
babies, whose future health will be determined not by the
whims of the microbes, but by how well or badly the people
treat their own bodies along the way.

CHAPTER 7

AIDS, Yuppie Flu and the Common Cold

Modern "scientific" medical practise relies very largely on medicines whose ultimate effect is to impair the patient's immune system.

This is no secret, no great discovery. It is discussed in all the relevant literature. But it has never seemed significant until today when the world is faced with an epidemic rooted in a pervasive crippling of the immune system. The drugs synthesized since the end of World War II have achieved their end—the antibiotic sterilization, more or less, of patients' bodies—at the expense of the immune system, and AIDS is the last stop on the line. The immune system cannot be undermined indefinitely without a price being paid. The chickens have come home to roost.

Harris L. Coulter Ph.D
(*AIDS & Syphilis: The Hidden Link*, 1987)

What do AIDS, yuppie flu, and the common cold have in common?

- They all reflect a state of diminished resistance to infection, in other words a state of lowered immuno-competence due to a weakened immune system and reduced vitality.
- They are all lifestyle-related problems insoluble by traditional medicine.

As immunocompetence depends on the maintenance of homeostasis within the body, and as homeostasis in turn depends on correct diet and other lifestyle factors, it again becomes clear that these health problems are caused, primarily, not by germs or viruses, but by wrong diet and other lifestyle factors, not the least of which factors is the use of medical drugs which further damage an already damaged immune system.

Most of the germs and viruses associated with the common cold, yuppie flu and AIDS reside acquiescently within the bodies of all people, all the time, in a form which is harmless; they are a normal part of our make up as they are in all animals. They change form to become pathogenic (harmful) only with the deterioration of the milieu surrounding them, ie the *milieu interieur*. For this reason the infections are referred to as opportunistic infections, "attacking" only when the opportunity is presented. These microbes appear in different forms, more or less in a predictable sequence according to the body's state of deterioration; thus a mild state of immunodeficiency may result in only a slight head cold, while a poorer state may result in a heavy cold or more chronic respiratory condition and so on. An even more run-down state of vitality will permit more infections to commence, such as candida, herpes, hepatitis and other symptoms which together are called a complex or a syndrome denoting the patient's overall condition; hence the terms AIDS-related complex (ARC) and chronic fatigue syndrome (CFS), the latter being one of a number of names for yuppie flu.

As in all areas of medicine, the subject appears to be more complicated than it really is, but despite all the confusing names there is in fact only one disease which is a toxic, out of balance, run-down *milieu interieur* in a body showing all the signs of it. This run-down state is a direct result of harmful habits, wrong diet, overwork, stress, late nights and so on which, according to degree, can soon reduce a vigorous young person to chronic fatigue and its associated syndrome. And if in addition to "respectable" bad habits, habits more outrageous to the body are indulged in—such as recreational drugs, continued sexual excesses, and the inevitable associated heavy use of antibiotics and other medical drugs—the body together with its immune system becomes reduced to tatters, additional life-threatening infections break out, and recovery may or may not be possible.

Thus it can be seen that AIDS (Acquired Immune Deficiency Syndrome) is no more than a downhill extension of a less serious syndrome, the so-called chronic fatigue syndrome, the entire show from start to finish being self-generated without the assistance of germs and viruses caught from someone else. That microbes from outside may or may not add to the problem is not disputed; the fact is they are not necessary.

Yuppie Flu

Yuppie flu is one of a number of names given to the condition of general malaise and fatigue accompanied by various troublesome infections which results when the body for one reason or another becomes chronically run down. The condition is known also as chronic fatigue syndrome and myalgic encephalomyelitis. The malaise of chronic fatigue was described in a book published in the 1920s called *Chronic Fatigue Intoxication* by Edward H. Ochsner, BS MD FACS, Professor of Clinical Surgery, University of Illinois, in which he described the connection between toxemia and the state of disease:

> "Long-continued, excessive use of narcotics and alcoholic stimulants favor its development."
>
> "That mental over-work and emotional over-stimulation are often contributory causes is quite evident."
>
> "The foundation for this affection is very frequently laid during the period of adolescence, the years when ambition is apt to run riot and when the wish and the will to do and dare far exceed the physical strength to execute."

"One of the most common combinations of causes is the combination of over-working and over-eating, when excessively fatigued, or severe exertion on a full stomach. These combinations so alter the end results of digestion that the pabulum which is absorbed acts as a mild poison instead of a true food."

"Ordinarily the body rapidly recuperates from moderately excessive fatigue but if this excessive exertion is persisted in day after day for a considerable period of time and particularly if the work is done at an abnormally high rate of speed, the point ultimately comes when the system becomes so supersaturated with fatigue material that it is no longer able to rid itself of this excessive accumulation."

Professor Ochsner went on to describe the types of people who most frequently suffer chronic fatigue and they are of course the very same types who have it today.

For many years the illness of chronic fatigue was thought by doctors to be in the minds of people who felt wretched without being able to display an obvious symptom, but since our more affluent and permissive lifestyle has led to the condition occurring more commonly and in more serious forms in which multiple infections are displayed, the illness has now been recognized as real.

A comparison of young peoples' lifestyles of fifty years ago and today clearly reveals the causes of "yuppie flu" and why today it is not just flu, not just fatigue, but a syndrome of associated problems. Fifty years ago most people, even if they had wanted to, could not afford to drink hard liquor, smoke tailormade cigarettes or dine in restaurants. Not many people drank much at all; no one except society people did these things or had wine with meals. Children took cut lunches to school and when thirsty they drank water. Nice girls—and that was just about all girls—never smoked, touched liquor or did anything more daring. Even Saturday night was not too late a night because hardly any young folk owned a car and the dances ended at 11:30 so people could catch the last train or bus home. No one had much money, so chronic fatigue was pretty well outside of peoples' financial resources. In fact, no one knew there was such a thing as chronic fatigue, let alone herpes, myalgic encephalomyelitis (ME), candida and things like that. Marijuana was thought to be the name of a Mexican dancing girl.

ME, yuppie flu, chronic fatigue syndrome or whatever else you want to call it is nothing more than a badly run-down state of the body which results in a depleted state of immunocompetence, and as this state is an acquired one, it becomes apparent that what is known as the chronic fatigue syndrome is different from AIDS only in matter of degree.

Apart from the factors of a "fast-living" lifestyle that lead to chronic fatigue syndrome, there are two additional factors that are probably more destructive to the body than all the others. They are: antibiotics and "recreational" drugs, the most common of the latter being marijuana. Whereas these drugs have been until recently regarded as fairly harmless, it is now known they are terribly destructive to the immune system. In regard to marijuana, a recent report reveals it to be, in the words of a scientist of pharmacology, a *devastating* drug that attacks and impairs the brain. Dr Gabriel Nahas, consultant to the UN Commission on Narcotics and Professor of Anaesthesiology at Columbia University, New York, said that marijuana was a sinister drug and much more devastating than doctors had thought, in view not only of its acute impairing properties but of its long-term toxic effects on lung and immune defences, brain and reproductive functions. Dr Nahas said studies had shown hashish smokers had six times the average incidence of schizophrenia, which was irreversible, and that children of mothers who smoked "pot" faced ten times the danger of developing leukemia. Put that in your pipe, man (but don't smoke it).

The syndrome of infections and other symptoms associated with chronic fatigue, most of which stem from within the body, include various forms of herpes, candida, glandular fever, hepatitis and chlamydia, which are often accompanied by swollen lymph glands, fevers, sweats, sore throats and other vague and not identified symptoms such as headaches and various aches and pains, all of which simply add up to the fact the body is sick right through. Thoroughly confused as to whether his patient has chronic fatigue syndrome, ME, glandular fever (infectious mononucleosis), or yuppie flu, which amount to the same thing anyway, the doctor mutters something about a virus, dispenses some more antibiotics out of pure habit, and hopes the patient won't get any worse. But antibiotics, besides being useless against viruses, are an immune suppressant and toxic in the body, so you can bet they will, in the long run, do more harm than good. They merely add another risk to an already risky lifestyle, if indeed they are not already implicated.

Glandular fever, sometimes called student's disease or kissing disease, is said to be transmissible to susceptible subjects by the Epstein–Barr virus. As well as being included in the range of complaints now known simply as ME it is also part of the AIDS-related complex (ARC) and of AIDS itself. It is characterized by the usual signs that accompany immunodeficiency such as fatigue, sore throat, headache, depression, enlarged lymph nodes, and abnormal lymphocytes in the blood.

However, a two-year study of patients with chronic fatigue syndrome at the University of Washington School of Medicine, reported in July 1990, concluded that no evidence could be found to support the hypothesis that chronic fatigue syndrome was caused by the Epstein–Barr virus or any other virus. What the researchers did find was that the "victims" "had a strikingly higher rate of lifetime and current major depression" than people without the syndrome. Once again it is important to realize that although depression may be a factor in causing the syndrome, it is just as likely that depression is, like the fatigue itself, just another of the symptoms. Thus, while it is logical to suspect an apparently common denominator to be the cause of a certain disease (such as the Epstein–Barr and other viruses associated with hepatitis, cancer, AIDS and so on), a more in-depth assessment reveals such viruses to be only effects and not causes, the real cause of disease being the disrupted homeostasis within the body.

As mentioned earlier, the common cold never occurs to people with proper homeostasis, even when concentrated virus solutions are squirted directly into their nostrils. With declining community health standards fewer and fewer people are capable of displaying such resistance to infections, a fact borne out by the increasing incidence to all kinds of infections, including rarer varieties such as malaria, Ross River fever, Lyme disease[1] and Legionnaire's disease.

Because many common bad lifestyle habits are accepted as normal and apparently harmless, and because their damaging effects are insidious and not clearly related to the lowered vitality they gradually cause, when the symptoms begin—fatigue, swollen glands, sore throat, headaches, etc—the lifestyle factors escape scrutiny and it is assumed some sort of germ or virus is responsible. The suspects, usually viruses but sometimes germs, are of course to be found, and association is often sufficient in the eyes of medical researchers to establish their guilt. So it is with another "up and coming" "disease" displaying headaches, sore throat, fevers, sweats, aches and pains, swollen lymph glands, chronic fatigue, etc, called Lyme disease[1], held to be caused by a spirochete (germ) picked up from a tick

---

[1] Lyme disease was named after the town of Lyme in Connecticut where the symptoms were first associated with tick bites. The belief is now widespread that a special spirochete germ from a special sort of tick is the cause of the disease, but this has never been proven. Other kinds of ticks are now said to be carriers of the germ and in Australia the bite of the common bush tick has eventuated in symptoms accepted to be Lyme disease. However, confusion exists in medical circles because not only do the ticks vary from place to place but so do the spirochetes. In Australia the spirochete allegedly carried by the bush tick has evaded detection altogether.

bite. However, millions of people get bitten by ticks without getting Lyme disease, just as it is possible to pick up the spirochete associated with syphilis without getting syphilis. Thus, while poison from a tick bite, with or without spirochetes, will obviously tend to impair the recipient's homeostasis, the ticks' participation should be looked upon as merely an additional factor in an already deteriorated situation.

In view of the confusion that has always existed about the association of germs and viruses with various disease conditions, including Lyme disease, one would wonder why medical research is still so firmly dedicated to the germ theory. It is interesting, however, that the blame for Lyme disease has been given (by association) to a germ (spirochete), and it is interesting too that Professor Luc Montagnier, the discoverer of HIV, now that he no longer believes HIV to be the cause of AIDS (*see* Chapter 8), believes a germ is involved. Will his germ, when he discovers it (which no doubt he will), resemble the spirochete of Lyme disease? Or perhaps one of the many germs that were blamed for beriberi?

AIDS-related Complex (ARC)

A complex means the same thing as a syndrome, which is a group of signs and symptoms that collectively indicate or characterize a disease or other abnormal condition.

When AIDS was first recognized as a more or less complete breakdown of the immune system and not merely the coincidental onset of a number of unrelated infections, much inquiry ensued to identify the reason for the breakdown. These inquiries revealed that preceding the syndrome of full-blown AIDS there occurred a lesser pattern of signs and symptoms like those of the chronic fatigue syndrome, which indicated the likely progression to AIDS; so to differentiate between the two conditions between which there was no clear demarcation, the lesser pattern was given the name of AIDS-related Complex (ARC). That

ARC was the same as the pattern of signs and symptoms appearing in the "straight" heterosexual world as chronic fatigue syndrome seemed not to be noticed, and so it was assumed they are separate illnesses. If you were heterosexual and presented with fatigue, headaches, candida, herpes and swollen lymph glands, the diagnosis would be chronic fatigue syndrome; if you were gay, the same symptoms would be diagnosed as ARC or even AIDS.

There are, of course, many pathways to the fatigue and malaise of chronic fatigue syndrome and ARC, which means they are not confined to any particular segment of society. Not only are yuppies and male homosexuals in the running, so too are students, teenagers, executives, playboys, doctors, housewives or anyone else one way or another overstressing their bodies.

But it is far worse for a homosexual person to be diagnosed with ARC than it is for a housewife to be diagnosed with chronic fatigue syndrome because ARC carries with it the implied sentence of death which can be as devastating as the bone-pointing ritual of the Aboriginals and which, together with further suppression of the immune system caused by subsequent medical treatment, as likely as not ensures progression to full AIDS.

That ARC does not necessarily mean further deterioration to AIDS is demonstrated by the many people with ARC (or chronic fatigue) who have stabilized their condition or, better still, have regained their health. The lifestyle factors which comprise the vicious spiral that leads to full AIDS are necessarily of a more damaging nature than those needed to cause ARC. As will be described later, these factors do not include the so-called AIDS virus, which has never been demonstrated, let alone proven, to cause AIDS, and in fact in many cases cannot even be detected.

AIDS: What It is Not

There are thousands of people in modern world countries and perhaps millions in third world countries who are thought to have AIDS simply because they "test positive" for the feared and supposedly deadly retrovirus called HIV. Most of these people are in average health, not displaying the sickness of the syndrome which is AIDS. So how on earth can someone without a syndrome be said to have the syndrome? AIDS is a syndrome and if you don't have the syndrome you don't have AIDS.

Moreover, even if it were true that HIV was the cause of AIDS, and this has never been more than supposition as will be shown, the fact that antibodies to the virus are detectable in someone's blood does not mean they harbor the virus at all; on the contrary, it means the same as in the case of all viruses, which is that the body has in the past encountered the virus and has mounted a defense against it.

That some of these HIV positive people, particularly those in the high-risk category (those busy destroying themselves), will eventually display AIDS is only to be expected, but that does not prove anything other than that their high-risk behavior is responsible, because it is a fact that even in the high-risk group, less than three per cent of "AIDS antibody positive" people have proceeded to develop "full blown" AIDS. And how many of these were taken over the brink by destructive medical procedures and the associated paranoid fear of their death sentence? The typical paranoia associated with the "deadly AIDS virus" was displayed on one occasion in Sydney when a policeman, bitten in a struggle with an AIDS suspect, later in abject fear shot himself dead with his own service pistol!

The Medical Definition of AIDS

There has been a great deal of confusion among doctors as to how to diagnose AIDS, and this is no wonder when it is considered that most of the information of the subject released by the so-called AIDS establishment is based on pure supposition. A virus is supposed to be the cause but can hardly ever be found; antibodies to the virus can be found in most cases but not in all cases. People with the antibodies mostly don't get sick while some without antibodies do. So, setting aside the theory of the virus as more or less irrelevant, the "official" method of diagnosis has been on the basis of whether a patient had one or more of the classic symptoms, such as pneumocystis pneumonia, Kaposi's sarcoma, cytomegalovirus, or others of the AIDS complex or chronic fatigue syndrome. As already mentioned, any of these could get you an AIDS pronouncement if you happened to be a male homosexual or an intravenous drug user, whereas for anyone else a diagnosis would be made in an unbiased fashion and be called simply pneumonia, hepatitis, or perhaps chronic fatigue.

As this method of diagnosis is at best only an "educated guess", a new system has been proposed by which a patient will be defined as having AIDS if their T4 (also called CD4) lymphocyte level falls below a certain figure. Thus, if and when this method is adopted, a person without a syndrome will be decreed to have the syndrome simply on this account, but even if at this stage the diagnosis is wrong, it won't be for long, because as fear takes hold and the destructive medical drugs get to work, the patient's already compromised immune system can only get worse. When fear alone (*see* reference which follows) can reduce a patient's normal T4 cell count by over fifty per cent, from 494 to 234 in one week, the new method of diagnosing AIDS would appear to be based on just as shaky a foundation as the "official" AIDS theory itself.

Medical "maverick" Dr Laurence Badgley of San Francisco has had as much experience personally helping AIDS patients as anybody, and is the author of two books about it, *Healing AIDS Naturally* and *Choose To Live*. About T4 cells he has this to say:

> "People with AIDS must learn that much of what they are told about AIDS is mere speculation, ie theories. The idea that the virus invades white blood cells, called T4 helper cells, and destroys them is

one such theory. This theory and myth has been presented to the public as fact. The idea that a diminished number of T4 cells is the critical factor in the development of AIDS is another such theory. The idea that a number of T4 cells below 200 is the magic measure of whether a person should start taking AZT is a pig-in-the-poke choice of numbers.

In my own medical practise I have a few patients who have had less than 50 T4 helper cells for months and years and they haven't become weakened or ill with serious infections. On the other hand one patient who followed a natural therapy had a T4 cell increase from less than 100, to over 600, at which time he developed pneumocystis carinii pneumonia.

T4 white blood cell counts are intimately related to mental focus. One of my patients was without symptoms and went to another doctor for an "AIDS test". The doctor did the test, which was positive, as well as the T4 helper cell count, which was 494 and normal. Upon learning that his antibody test was positive, the patient went into a tailspin of depression and fear. One week later he returned to the doctor because of his anxiety, and his T4 helper cell count was taken again. After one week of depression and no other symptoms his T4 cell count fell over 50% to 234.

This intimate relationship of the mind and body raises a question about the true nature of the AIDS epidemic. It is not far fetched to postulate that much of the immune system depression among AIDS-test-positive patients might be the result of doctors telling them that it is likely they will get AIDS and die. The brain is a giant immune system gland that operates on hope, joy, and optimism. The gland turns off in response to mental attitudes of fear and depression.

The question is raised as to how many people are dying because they have been programmed to die. The observation is made that doctors who tell their patients they have a terminal disease are programming their patients to die. The charge is made that these doctors are performing malpractise."

A current news item reports that Australian hepatitis experts at Sydney's Westmead Hospital are currently agitating for speeded up approval for a new "breakthrough drug" for hepatitis C. The drug is called alpha interferon, and according to "eminent medical researchers" it has proved very successful, "the preliminary results showing that 65% of hepatitis C patients have responded excellently to it"[2] and that "some 25 to 40% of sufferers are potentially cured". The side effects included depression, skin rashes and low white blood cell counts.

Those people at risk of hepatitis C, said the experts, were intravenous drug users, people receiving blood transfusions, renal dialysis patients, people who have been tattooed and male homosexuals. But aren't these the people who are also vulnerable to AIDS? Could it be—the question arises again—that AIDS experts, yuppie flu experts and hepatitis experts are all trying to solve the same problem? That the "different" diseases they specialize in are, in fact, all only slightly different symptoms of the one disease?

Whether you agree or not, pay attention to this paragraph of the report: "Professor Farrell said alpha interferon did have side-effects but they could be managed. Serious side-effects—in about five percent of patients—were *depression, skin rashes and a low white blood cell count*" (author's italics). What is meant by "they could be managed"? Does this mean that "high-risk" patients whose

---

[2] This percentage of favorable reactions is the typical percentage gained by the placebo effect in all kinds of diseases, and in the absence of controlled studies cannot be attributed to anything other than the placebo effect. In chronic disease, the immense power of the placebo effect—both for good and sometimes for bad—cannot be overestimated (*see* "The Mental Factor" in Chapter 16).

symptom—hepatitis—is one of the pre-AIDS symptoms, will be given a drug which will add more AIDS symptoms? Lower their white cell count?

What if their white cell count hits the magic 200 level?[3] Will they be plucked out of the hepatitis category and put in the AIDS category? Given AZT?

The blind leading the blind is not malpractice, but it is just as sad to behold.

AIDS: What It is

AIDS is a state of illness characterized by depleted vitality and a progressive increase in severity of a number of opportunistic infections, all of which are associated with a more or less complete breakdown of the immune system. The name AIDS is an acronym standing for Acquired Immune Deficiency Syndrome, and although this title accurately describes as well the condition called chronic fatigue syndrome (the two syndromes differing only in degree), it is applied only to the more severe, more or less final stage. Again it must be made clear that the mere trace of a suspected viral infection (HIV or any other virus) does not constitute AIDS, nor does it mean that AIDS will develop.

None of the infections which together constitute AIDS are new to medicine; what makes AIDS a "new" disease, just as ME and chronic fatigue syndrome are "new", is the unusual appearance of a number of the symptoms at the same time or in close succession. That chronic fatigue syndrome and AIDS are "new diseases" is not because new strains of viruses have evolved, it is because *a new lifestyle has evolved*, availing to an already semi-sick society the additional potential for destruction: permissiveness, junk food, promiscuity, and a bewildering array of drugs both medicinal and "recreational"—a lifestyle reminiscent of

---

[3] Currently the AIDS establishment recommends that AZT be given at levels below 500!

that which led to the decline and fall of ancient Rome, only using drugs instead of wine.

The evidence that medical drugs are a major, if not *the* major, factor in AIDS is overwhelming. Dr Joan McKenna, Director of Research, T&M Associates, Berkeley, California, has researched AIDS since 1981. She began by searching all the medical literature of the past for reports of illnesses displaying AIDS-like symptoms.

One report she found was on an epidemic of pneumocystis carinii pneumonia (PCP) among children in European orphan asylums after World War II after the children had been given penicillin and terramycin to protect them from infections. PCP is one of the classic symptoms of AIDS and is the main denominator in AIDS diagnosis. Pneumocystis carinii exists dormantly in all healthy humans and becomes pathological only when the immune system is selectively damaged.

The outbreak of PCP among the orphans was not due to contagion but due to the individual damage caused to the children's immune systems by the very drugs designed to protect them.

Thus it became evident to Dr McKenna that the habitual prolific use of antibiotics by some homosexuals was the main common factor among all the factors involved in AIDS.

In reviewing the medical histories of 100 homosexual men, Dr McKenna noted the most common problems encountered by them were:

- *Gonorrhea*—multiple incidents, up to twenty a year, treated with antibiotics.
- *Hepatitis*—high incidence, some chronic.
- *Non-specific urethritis*—multiple incidents, sometimes chronic, perhaps six or seven episodes a year, with increasing doses of antibiotics as antibiotics became less effective,
- *Dermatological eruptions*—treated by continuous use of antibiotics, tetracycline and corticosteroids for five to eighteen years.

- *Psychological conditions*—for which were taken sedatives, tranquillizers and mood drugs.
- *Chronic sore throat*—more than fifty per cent reported frequent episodes treated by antibiotics.
- *Herpes simplex*—twenty-five per cent reported chronic herpes, ninety per cent herpes within the past ten years.
- *Allergies*—high incidences both chronic and severe treated by allergy medications and symptomatic suppressants.
- *Lymphadenopathy*—frequent to chronic swollen lymph glands in forty per cent of cases.
- *Diarrhea*—high incidence, various treatments.
- *Recreational drugs*—nearly universal use of marijuana, multiple and complex use of LSD, MDA, PCP, heroin, cocaine, amyl and butyl nitrites, amphetamines, barbituates, ethyl chloride, opium, mushrooms and "designer drugs".

Dr McKenna said that out of the 100 men, one fourth shared nine or more of these conditions, and the only ones out of the 100 diagnosed as having AIDS or ARC all came from this smaller group.

Dr McKenna went on to describe the grotesque damaging effects of the various antibiotics and added that although "recreational" drugs such as marijuana, cocaine, "poppers", etc are all immunosuppressive and therefore major co-factors in AIDS, "they should not deflect attention from therapeutic drugs *whose immunosuppressive impact, all in all, is probably far greater*".

The dangers associated with antibiotics have long been known, but this knowledge has not prevented careless and prolific use of them in the treatment of patients who are totally unaware of the dangers. In 1975 Dr Maynard Murray, MD B.Sc,[4] of Fort Myers, Florida and a practising physician

---

[4] Quotation taken from Dr Murray's book *Sea Energy Agriculture* (1976). Dr Murray: Bachelor of Science 1934; Medical degree 1936; University of Cincinnati plus five and a half years' post-graduate study of internal medicine and ear, nose and throat specialty. Taught and directed experiments at University of Cincinnati from

and physiologist for forty-five years, said in his book *Sea Energy Agriculture* (Valentine Books, 1976):

> "Despite drug industry propaganda, these new medicines are fraught with shortcomings, and the long-term effects may prove them more harmful than beneficial.
>
> Dr Finland and his colleagues recently examined Boston Hospital records covering a period of 24 years in order to evaluate the long-term results of wonder drug therapy. They learned that wonder drugs had reduced the death rate from infection caused by pneumococci and streptococci, but there had been *an increase in deaths due to infection from bacteria which previously were considered harmless.* [This is what happens with AIDS.] Reliance on antibiotics to combat infectious diseases is to live in a fool's paradise, noted Dr Finland."

The measure of damage to the immune system by which the progression of AIDS is assessed, apart from the obvious symptoms, is the count of white T cells in the blood; the lower the T cell count, the poorer the outlook.

[4] *continued*

1937–47, thereafter in private practice. Convinced that faulty nutrition was the major factor in human disease, Dr Murray reasoned that trace minerals deficient in the soil existed plentifully in fresh seawater, having been leached there from the land by rainwater over the centuries.

After forty years of experiments using seawater in carefully measured amounts as fertilizer, he proved his beliefs by showing that his experimental crops produced superior health in animals of all kinds. Possibly the most significant result was with a strain of mice which, because they usually develop breast cancer, are used in cancer research. When fed in accordance with Dr Murray's principles these mice did not develop cancer and maintained sound health and good condition to an advanced age.

It is the common belief that the diminution of the white cells is entirely due to the predatory activity of a virus which, it has been theorized (but never demonstrated), enters the white T cells and destroys them, so greatly damaging the immune system. This belief, held worldwide, began with the hastily formed opinion of a single researcher employed by the US National Institute of Health, Dr Robert Gallo, and this opinion, still not formulated into a plausible theory—let alone proven—is why the entire world fears a virus which has never been shown to destroy white cells in the human body and which in many cases of AIDS cannot even be detected.

Research has disclosed that in only fifty per cent of AIDS patients can active HIV be detected, and even when it can be detected, only 1 in 10,000 white cells shows signs of it at most, and sometimes only 1 in 100,000 cells. Fewer than 1 in 500 of a host's T cells contain even dormant HIV. Obviously if a patient has no HIV present you cannot blame it for destroying the white cells. Furthermore, assuming HIV is harmful to white cells in the body (and to repeat: this has never been demonstrated), if it inhabits only 1 in 10,000 white cells it could never kill enough of them to remotely approach the body's normal capacity to make new ones. As the world's leading virologist, Professor Peter Duesberg of the University of California, said recently: "The idea of a virus killing so few cells and by so doing killing the body, is like trying to conquer China by shooting five Chinese soldiers a day." Impossible.

However, there is a simple watertight explanation of why AIDS patients display diminished numbers of T cells and in some cases none at all: long-term destructive living habits, especially the use of drugs—including medicinal drugs—so overtax the immune system that the thymus is gradually destroyed, and as the thymus is the only source of new T cells in the body, when the old T cells wear out there can be no new ones to replace them. An additional demolishing effect on the immune system and specifically destructive to the thymus is severe emotional stress, an illustration of which has already been given. Autopsies of

AIDS patients show that in every case the thymus is severely atrophied or destroyed.[5]

That explanation being correct, the question arises why do some children have AIDS? To answer that it must be emphasized that a lot of people are said to have AIDS simply because they test positive to HIV antibodies. This is not AIDS, nor does it mean AIDS is likely. To repeat, AIDS is a syndrome of infections which have nothing to do with viral antibodies. Children with real AIDS are born with defective immune systems, usually of mothers who are, or have been, drug addicts. Hemophiliacs, no matter how "clean-living", are at risk of AIDS because for a start they have been born with defective systems and throughout life are compelled to suffer the constant trauma of blood transfusions and the associated constant trauma of medicinal drugs, the combined effects of which over a long period are destructive to the immune system. Even transplant patients on immunosuppressing drugs to prevent tissue rejection of their new organs frequently display AIDS-like symptoms, which only makes sense— if you set out to depress the immune system what would you expect?

Although it had been observed by some doctors for a good number of years, AIDS first attracted the attention of the US medical profession in about 1981, not long after the advent of the "gay liberation", and because most of the new cases were male homosexuals it became known as "the gay disease". Gay liberation was a follow-on to

[5] The *New England Journal of Medicine* on 6 January contained a report (Hersch, Reuben, Rios et al) on ten homosexuals, eight relatively healthy and two with signs of AIDS. All had had multiple bouts of sexually transmitted diseases (STD) and associated medical treatment, all had used recreational drugs, and all had T cell ratio reversal as well as abnormal levels of thymus hormones, suggestive of thymus dysfunction or failure. At the American Association for the Advancement of Science meeting in June 1983, scientists reported that autopsies of twelve homosexuals who died of AIDS showed their thymus glands to be almost totally destroyed.

the permissive society of the 1960s and 70s in which it
became fashionable in all stratas of society to indulge in
promiscuous sex, recreational drugs, junk food and fast
living. When gays were "freed" and lost a lot of their
inhibitions, some of them went wild. In the cities where
they congregated, gay bars opened, then gay discos and
gay "bath houses". In these places some homosexuals
indulged in the most unbelievably promiscuous sexual
behavior, sustained by chemical drugs, marijuana, alcohol,
etc, performed over and over to exhaustion, and it was *only
from this sub-group* of homosexuals—the ones most
dissipated and depleted—that AIDS took its toll. This fact
was obvious right from the start when the Center of Disease
Control (CDC) conducted its first investigation into AIDS,
long before the HIV theory was concocted. The most
outstanding factor common to AIDS patients, the CDC
noted, was that they were all far more sexually active than
the average (about four times as much) with a
correspondingly intense history of medical treatment.

Anal sex is acknowledged to be a major factor in AIDS
and the official explanation for this is that the delicate
membranes of the human anus are more easily permeable
by the HIV than are the membranes of the female vagina,
and this, say the "experts", is also the reason why the AIDS
virus has not spread much into the heterosexual world.
This explanation is, however, absurd, because leaving
membranes right out of it—if ninety-five per cent of
homosexual AIDS patients are of the anal receptive
persuasion,[6] why did not the person who gave them the
virus get AIDS too? The dominant partner in the anal sex
act must have HIV himself in order to inject it into his
passive partner, so why are so few dominant partners

---

[6] Among 400 consecutive homosexuals screened for AIDS in South
Florida at the Institute of Tropical Medicine, Miami, between
January and November 1983, Doctors Mark Whiteside and Carole
MacLeod found that the only ones who had symptoms of AIDS
or ARC were the "receivers" or "passive partners" in anal inter-
course.

affected? The answer obviously has nothing to do with HIV.

The reason that the dominant homosexual sex partners are far less prone to AIDS than the anal receptive passive partners is that their behavior is less destructive to their immune systems. They tend to have different personalities, they rely less on drugs, and they are incapable of the wanton promiscuity so weakening to the body, whereas the passive partners tend to indiscriminately use chemical drugs such as poppers (amyl nitrite and butyl nitrite) to enhance their sexual highs and to relax their anal muscles. While the dominant partners cannot physically be so promiscuous and avoid the use of drugs that will prevent them achieving an erection, the anal receptive partners, not being so restricted, can be far more promiscuous, having numerous sexual contacts with different partners every day. A survey of over 1000 male homosexuals, described in the *Spada Report* (James Spada, Signet Books, 1979), throws more light on this subject. The majority of homosexuals interviewed were promiscuous in varying degrees, and while some preferred always the dominant role in sex and some the passive role, most of them indulged in both. However, some gays gained so much extraordinary pleasure from the passive role that they indulged in it with as many partners as they could, as often as they could, and it is significant that so many from this sub-group came down with AIDS. This sexual high of the passive partner is achieved by the physical stimulation of the prostate gland which produces an orgasm of "out of this world" intensity and which is greatly prolonged, variously described as "absolutely mind blowing", "volcanic", "fabulous", etc and which leaves the subject mentally and physically absolutely drained. As if this sort of behavior wasn't weakening enough, it is also known that some of the anal lubricants used by anal receptive gays are immunosuppressive when absorbed into the bloodstream, as has been shown to be the case with sperm in the anal canal.

In addition to such wanton behavior are the further

immunosuppressive effects of medical drugs, antibiotics, etc which are liberally prescribed by doctors to "control" the many infections and sexually transmitted diseases common among promiscuous people. Antibiotics are particularly damaging to the immune system and it is no wonder AIDS progresses rapidly once a certain point is reached, particularly when the bone-pointing death sentence of AIDS is pronounced and the deadly AZT[7] chemotheraphy is commenced.

The pronounced immunosuppressing effect of semen injected into the anal canal has been traced by Dr Richard Ablin of State University, New York, to the enzyme transmutamenase contained in semen and, apart from animal experiments to demonstrate this, there is additional evidence that the high incidence of AIDS among hemophiliacs is due to the same enzyme contained in the drug Factor VIII, upon which hemophiliacs constantly depend. In *Lancet*, April 1985, Dr Ablin wrote:

> Association is not proof of cause, and agents such as HIV may turn out to be passengers on an already sinking ship. It would be reasonable to postulate some other transmissible agent, even a non-infectious one, which contributes to immune dysfunction and possibly predisposes to opportunistic infections . . . As an alternative to the hypothesis that AIDS is solely an infectious disease I suggest that the opportunistic infections and tumors such as Kaposi's sarcoma seen in AIDS patients result from a combination of lifestyle hazard and immuno-deficiency, whereas in patients with hemophilia the infections are a consequence of immunosuppression resulting from infusion of anti-hemophiliac factor.

To what extent semen is a major factor in AIDS has not been determined, but the fact that it is a factor certainly helps to explain the predominant role of receptive anal

---

[7] *See* the statements by Duesberg and McKenna in the addendum to Chapter 8, and also "AZT" in Chapter 9.

sex in the disease. It has of course been pointed out that anal sex has been practised widely in some communities for centuries with no reported ill effects, which is true, but never in history have anal receptive sex partners received such amounts of semen so constantly, accompanied by so many drugs, as since the advent of gay bath houses, and it is a fact that the cities in which AIDS first appeared are the very cities in which bath houses first appeared.

Of course, only a relatively small proportion of all homosexuals are so neurotically drawn to outrageously treat their bodies by what in the AIDS business is called "high-risk behavior", and therefore the majority of homosexuals, HIV positive or not, need have no more fear of AIDS than the average heterosexual, which fact is already being borne out by the steady decline in AIDS cases among them. The decline is not because gays are using condoms or clean hypodermics, it is because the majority of the "high-risk" gays have either already perished or have wised up and moderated their behavior. This fact cannot now be disputed, given the large number of previous AIDS patients, homosexual and heterosexual, who have regained good health by adopting a better lifestyle, just as have other so-called incurables in the past overcome cancer, leukemia, MS and other "terminal" diseases.

Thus it can be seen that AIDS is not the slightest threat to anybody providing they do not debilitate their bodies with drugs, malnutrition and other high-risk behavior and, if they clean up their lifestyle really well, nor will they need fear the other so-called terminal diseases. The great AIDS epidemic, predicted year after year by the virusmongers, simply has not happened, not because people are practising "safe sex" or using condoms, but because still only relatively few people are living dangerously enough to completely destroy their immune systems.

That drugs of all kinds are the bottom line in the drama of AIDS was pretty clear right at the beginning, but the fact was obscured due to incompetent data recording. Because it was clear that intravenous drug users were getting AIDS as well as homosexuals, the patients were divided on the records as being in one or the other of these categories, which did not allow for the many cases where homosexuals fell into both categories, and because such patients were listed only in the homosexual category the impression was given that drugs were not implicated at all in that great number of cases. But not only that, no drugs other than intravenous drugs were even mentioned. There seemed to be not the vaguest notion that other drugs can be every bit as dangerous, but when all drugs are taken into account, including alcohol, marijuana and the other countless recreational drugs, plus the antibiotics, etc taken by the cartload, the fact emerges loud and clear that the indiscriminate use of drugs is the number one AIDS factor. That the constant use of medical drugs alone can cause AIDS is illustrated by the case of a heterosexual doctor in San Francisco who came down with AIDS through his addiction to medical drugs. Fortunately by completely changing his lifestyle and abandoning all drugs he averted imminent death and made a fine recovery.[8]

Why the "AIDS Establishment" based in the Center of Disease Control, US National Institute of Health (CDC & NIH) holds on to its hysterical belief in the virus theory of AIDS is incomprehensible—assuming its members are sincere—because the true story is as clear as the nose on your face and has been for a long time. As far back as 1968, AIDS was starting to appear among drug addicts. In that year Professor Gordon Stewart of Tulane University in New Orleans commenced a three-year study of drug addiction in New Orleans and New York City. He reported that the drug addicts suffered all kinds of opportunistic infections—eighty-five to ninety per cent of them had hepatitis to some degree. He said they were emaciated with "various weird blood-born infections" together with candida and cryptococci. Darrell Yates Rist, New York journalist and AIDS researcher reported: "The intravenous drug users were in the lead, and only later the gays picked

---

[8] Refer to *Roger's Recovery from AIDS* by Dr Robert Owen, Davar Press, Malibu, California, 1987.

it up. The first case of AIDS I know of in the US was in 1976 when the baby of an IV drug user died of pneumocystis in San Francisco."

Dr Joseph Sonnabend of New York City made similar observations. He said:

> "I was seeing patients with a whole range of problems for years before AIDS came along. Swollen lymph glands, bladder problems, bowel problems of course. I was telling them this was going to lead to some major problem though I didn't know what. People would come in for treatment for gonorrhoea, get their shot of penicillin and go straight back to the bath houses to have sex again. They'd do that ten times a year. Of course there were going to be problems. One of my promiscuous patients would already have hepatitis B, hepatitis A, syphilis, gonorrhoea, cytomegalovirus, herpes simplex, Epstein-Barr virus."

A novel published in 1978, *Faggots* by Larry Kramer, described the typical behavior of some of the big city gays who indulged in orgies of drugs and sexual perversion almost every day, some of them averaging twenty or more sexual acts a week. The author described fifty-six different drugs used indiscriminately for kicks, and these did not include intravenous drugs or medicinal ones. All of them were immunosuppressive, all of them were associated with promiscuity.

That drugs, chemicals and junk food have become a normal, everyday part of life in some social circles is illustrated by an account in the book *Herpes, Cause and Control* by Dr William Wickett (Pinnacle Books, 1982):

> "We even took care of Max, a Hell's Angels type who was referred to us by the Venereal Disease Clinic. He had been treated there twice for syphilis and innumerable times for gonorrhea. He now had herpes. Max also admitted to having been addicted to heroin in the past, to smoking two packs of

cigarettes a day, to taking amphetamines and
sedatives, and to being a regular user of marijuana,
usually in combination with large quantities of
beer.

There was no mistake, Max had herpes
genitalis. There were blisters along the length of
the penis and several more on the scrotum.

But, alas, Max withdrew from our study. When
we explained we were testing a new drug, one from
which we had seen almost no side-effects, he
declined. Said he, 'I don't want to put anything
in my body that might be harmful.' "

Although at present the greatest number of people
with AIDS (PWA) in the USA are still male homosexuals,
the highest incidence of new cases is among young drug-
addicted heterosexuals in New York City, and in Australia
the highest incidence is among poorly situated Aboriginals
in Northern Queensland who, like hapless teenagers
abandoned by society with little hope for the future, seek
solace in drugs, liquor and junk food.

If HIV were necessary to cause AIDS, how on earth
did it find its way to north Queensland, there to selectively
attack a group of underprivileged Aboriginals and nobody
else? Is it mere coincidence that these Aboriginals practise
a self-destructive lifestyle similar in many ways to the self-
destructive lifestyles of other people with AIDS?

Having described the lifestyle factors that lead to the
end state of physical degeneration called AIDS, it must
be emphasized that AIDS is no more a fatal disease than
any other disease of civilization, including cancer,
providing corrective steps are taken before damage becomes
irreparable. HIV has absolutely no effect on a healthy body;
any harm it may cause is entirely by fear implanted in
the patient's mind by doctors brainwashed by the deluded
"authorities" in the US AIDS "establishment".

Dr Laurence Badgley has seen AIDS patients die, but
he has also seen them recover, and to repeat the last part
of the quote from his book *Healing AIDS Naturally*: "The

question is raised as to how many people are dying because they have been programmed to die. The observation is made that doctors who tell their patients they have a terminal disease are programming their patients to die. The charge is made that these doctors are performing malpractise.''

"Brainwashing" is a potent force, and most people have heard of how primitive Australian Aboriginals can punish one of their tribe with death simply by the ritual of "bone pointing". The capacity of the mind[9] to influence metabolic processes within the body for good or evil exists within everybody, primitive or educated, and a classic case of self-inflicted "bone pointing" is described in a book on psychotherapeutics by Dr Arthur Hallam of England, *The Key to Perfect Health* published in 1912:

> "But perhaps the most extraordinary case in point was furnished a few years ago by a late member of the medical profession, Dr Richardson, whose death was due to his own mental influence—he thought himself to death. He sustained injuries which were not serious, by falling off his bicycle, and he might easily have recovered from them if he had not taken up a feverish idea that they would produce lockjaw. He was progressing favorably when he announced to a brother physician that he would have lockjaw during the week and would die of it on the following Sunday. Despite all attempts to persuade him that the idea was absurd, he insisted on being treated with anti-toxins. If this had any effect at all, it seemed to increase the power of his imagination, and as a result, he developed alarming symptoms on the Thursday, and it became clear he would not recover. He died on the day he appointed, and of lockjaw, as he had predicted! He thought himself to death!
>
> The case is remarkable, not because it is rare for people to "think themselves to death", for they are doing so every day of the year, but because the

---

[9] *See* "The Mental Factor" in Chapter 15.

victim was a physiologist, supposedly reinforced by special training in the effects of the mind on the body. This training did not save him, but, as the evidence suggests, it made him worse. Mimetic disease killed him, and everything he knew of physiology helped to kill him."

Finally, emphasis must be added to the warning of the harmful effects of the useless anti-HIV medical drugs such as AZT, which alone are capable of destroying a functional immune system and, when added to the effects of the HIV bone-pointing ritual, remove all hope of recovery. Death of course will be blamed on HIV, and the drug companies will claim credit for having kept the patient alive for a while. With "friends" like that, who needs enemies?

Clearly the HIV theory of AIDS is wrong, and clearly Dr Richard Ablin is right: HIV when it can be found in people with AIDS is only a passenger on an already sinking ship. It is a mistake to accept that the ship cannot be saved; people with AIDS and the doctors who treat them have made enough mistakes already. The HIV theory, never tested, never proven, has degenerated from a bad mistake into a monumental farce, and the following chapter describes how it came about.

CHAPTER 8

The Myth of the AIDS Virus

Necessity is the mother of invention.
Anon. from old Latin

In democratic law a suspect is held to be innocent until proven guilty. A suspect may be held for questioning by police, but unless there is sufficient evidence against him he cannot even be brought to trial; he must be presumed innocent and released. To have been at the scene of the crime, acting in a suspicious manner, only marks a person as a suspect. To gain a conviction the prosecutor must show that the suspect actually committed the crime; the prosecutor must prepare a case and at the trial present evidence to prove it. There have been trials when the jury has been swayed by the oratory of the prosecutor and have found the accused guilty on flimsy evidence, and there have been other cases when the accused has been "framed" and found guilty on the strength of fabricated false evidence.

Science, like civil law, demands the truth; it is concerned only with cold, hard fact. All claims of new knowledge, new discoveries, must be supported by clear-cut, demonstrable data. Anecdotal evidence or speculation, no matter how convincing, is unacceptable until proven by exact scientific method. But even that is not enough. To gain full acceptance, a claim must not only pass scrutiny for publication in one or more scientific publications, it must then pass the scrutiny of all the scientific people who read the journals.

To prove that a specific germ (or virus) is guilty of causing a certain disease, the first thing a researcher must do is to ensure Koch's postulates (*see* Chapter 6) are satisfied, the first and most obvious of which is that in every case of the disease the accused germ must be present in significant numbers. If in only one case the germ cannot be detected at all, it obviously cannot be the cause. But that is only the beginning—even if the germ is detected in all cases it still doesn't mean that it has caused the disease, because there may be other germs also present in all cases, as happens in beriberi (*see* Chapter 6). So to make sure, Koch's second, third and fourth postulates must be met.

Koch's postulates have been discussed already, but whatever you may think of them one thing is certain: no germ or virus can infect a person's body from a distance; to do so it must necessarily be present in the body, it must be present in significant numbers, and it must be seen to be doing something.

Ever since germs were found to play a part in disease there have been many different germs identified to be associated with different disease conditions. As previously mentioned, some of these germs (and viruses) were proven capable of transmitting a particular disease and some were proven to be only incidental, but even the ones found guilty could not pass Koch's third postulate until the postulate was changed to admit susceptibility was a prerequisite for the germ to have effect. Thus it is accepted that for any germ or virus to do harm to anybody, that person must first of all be susceptible, which means that the real cause of any infectious disease is whatever it is that lowers a person's resistance.

AIDS is now considered to be a disease in its own right, characterized by the occurrence of multiple infections, none of them new. In the past when any one of these infections appeared on its own, which was rare, conventional drug treatment was employed and no mention made of immune deficiency. So AIDS has in fact done the world a service in that it has forced the medical profession to relax its vendetta against germs and viruses and focus instead on the real issue—susceptibility—or, in other words, immune deficiency.

Whereas the doctors of the 19th Century can be excused for not identifying the mysterious causes of beriberi, pellagra, etc, the immune-depressing factors of AIDS stand out like neon signs on a dark night and there can be no excuse other than blindness for ignoring them. But medicine is not really an art or a science, it is a commercially oriented industry, based on germs and drugs and more lately on viruses. So when AIDS appeared, medical research was myopically directed in search of the ultimate virus, one which is not governed by the laws of Nature, one which does not wait for someone's resistance to lower, but instead goes out and lowers it all on its own.

So urgent was the need for this discovery that a fair amount of invention had to be employed and a lot of conventional rules set aside. Formalities usually rigid and considered essential were dispensed with entirely, but this was no problem for Dr Robert Gallo because he worked for the US Government in the prestigious National Institute of Health. So in 1984 a new virus, unlike any other known, was announced, and became instantly famous as the AIDS virus. But so hurried was Dr Gallo to beat his French rivals, the announcement was the most premature in medical history. There were no medical trials, no double-blind studies, no epidemiological studies, no submissions to scientific journals, no scientific scrutiny or peer review. Not one of Koch's postulates were met and no proof has ever been produced.

When the subject of scientific accuracy was raised with Dr Gallo in an interview by Charles Ortleib, publisher of *The New York Native*, Mr Ortlieb reported Dr Gallo's response thus: "Dr Gallo told me that his early assertion that HIV is the cause of AIDS was not based purely on scientific grounds, but rather that he needed to bring the field to another extreme. Otherwise, he felt that people would be confused by multifactorial or crackpot theories.

I told him that I thought it was dangerous to mix his public health concerns with his statements of scientific truths. But, he insisted that he had the medical authority to do so."

Dr Gallo, who has since admitted the virus was not his discovery as he first claimed, refuses any debate on the matter of proof, while at the same time the man who originally discovered the virus, Dr Luc Montagnier, has announced his disbelief that HIV causes AIDS.

The case for HIV causing AIDS does not hold water, and in a court of law would be thrown out in very short time.

When germs were discovered in the 19th Century they were suspected to be the cause of most human diseases. And when viruses were discovered later on they automatically became the suspects in all the diseases that could not be blamed on germs. Early in this century when cancer research was speeding up, it was demonstrated at the Rockefeller Institute for Medical Research that a type of cancer peculiar to chickens could be transmitted from one susceptible chicken to another, and this led many researchers to suspect viruses to be the cause of all cancers and that cancer was contagious. This was never shown to be the case, but when President Nixon in his 1971 State of the Union address officially declared war on cancer in the belief that the sort of technology that split the atom and put man on the moon must surely succeed, research was again directed at viruses.

The war against cancer was directed by the US Government National Cancer Institute (NCI), a subsidiary of the US National Institute of Health. Totally committed to the belief in orthodox allopathic medicine and heavily influenced by the pharmaceutical companies, the research efforts of the National Cancer Institute achieved nothing despite the prodigious outlay in money, and it was eventually admitted that the war against cancer was lost. However, it was concluded once again that cancer was not caused by a virus.

With the advent of the AIDS epidemic among

homosexuals in the early 1980s, government health officials, having just lost the war on cancer, now found themselves with another war on their hands, one which they were determined to win. The research personnel were already there and lost no time switching from cancer research to research on AIDS. Dr Robert Gallo, head of the Laboratory of Human Cell Biology at the NCI, had been in charge of the NCI's war against cancer and was retained in charge for the war against AIDS. He even had a new virus that showed promise, a sort of left-over from the cancer research.

In his previous research into cancer, Gallo had discovered a new virus his team had isolated from the T cells of leukemia patients which he called Human T cell Leukemia Virus I and which he believed to be the cause of their leukemia. When epidemiological evidence on 600,000 test subjects (Japanese) showed this virus, HTLVI, to have absolutely no bearing on leukemia at all, Gallo maintained his stance that it could, but that the virus probably had a very long "latency period" of maybe forty years. As the latency period, ie the time between infection and symptoms, of viruses is usually measured in days, Gallo was either joking or trying out for the Guinness Book of Records.

In the following year, 1982, Gallo and his team discovered a new retro-virus they called HTLVII which came from a young man with hairy cell leukemia,[1] but this virus proved to be blameless and the team turned their virus-hunting efforts on to resolving the AIDS problem.

Convinced still that viruses were man's greatest enemy, Gallo set out to show that his HTLVI, if not the cause of leukemia, would prove to be the cause of AIDS. This was an odd change of opinion because having first said the virus caused an increase in white cells (leukemia), he was now saying it caused the decrease in white cells which is AIDS.

[1] *See The Health Revolution*, Chapter 2, in which the case is described by a Perth engineer who by dietary means completely cleared himself of hairy cell leukemia in a few months.

Early in 1983, Professor Luc Montagnier and his team of virologists at the Pasteur Institute in Paris were also searching for a virus they suspected of causing AIDS, and they found one. Tests done on a thirty-three-year old male homosexual who was promiscuous and who had AIDS symptoms revealed a novel retro-virus isolated from a lymph node, which Montagnier named lymphodenopathy-associated virus (LAV). He did not at that time claim it to be the cause of AIDS.

Montagnier's LAV, a sample of which was sent to Gallo in America, resembled Gallo's HTLVI but tests showed it to be distinctly different. Gallo continued in his assertions that HTLVI would prove to be the cause of AIDS, but at the same time he was cultivating in his laboratory the LAV from Montagnier's sample.

In December 1983 Gallo received a laboratory report on thirty-three blood samples from AIDS patients which showed thirty-one to be negative for viruses, the other two showing positive for LAV, not HTLVI. Thus if any virus was involved with AIDS at all, it had to be Montagnier's LAV.

But finding a virus was meaningless if, as in Gallo's two leukemia suppositions, the virus could not be shown to be doing something. But again this detail did not worry Gallo; he merely, as he had done before, assumed guilt by association. There was no time to spare, and Gallo was intent on beating his French rivals in the race to conquer AIDS, even if it meant ignoring the established research protocols.

It is normal procedure in scientific research that when new discoveries are made and conclusions arrived at, the research data is formally submitted to one or more reputable scientific or medical journals for review, and if accepted and published the data is assessed by all the experts. Following this initial step, months of discussion and argument usually ensue before general consensus is reached as to whether the concept is practical, useful and safe. This is traditional scientific and medical procedure.

In the case of Gallo's HIV hypothesis, all rules were

set aside. Gallo was the big chief, full of confidence, and he was backed by the US Government. Protocol was ignored, and instead of the HIV hypothesis appearing tentatively in some respectable medical journal, it was announced, fully fledged as a fait accompli, in two national newspapers, the *Wall Street Journal* and the *Washington Post*. That these two newspapers cater to the centers of the country's financial and political power itself arouses suspicions in what was going on. Why were the *New York Times* and the *San Francisco Examiner* not in on it? Be that as it may, it was only several days later, on 19 April 1984, that Gallo's formal announcement appeared in the *New Scientist*.[2] The report made no mention of Montagnier's LAV; instead, Gallo claimed he had discovered another altogether new virus called HTLVIII which he stated without fear of contradiction to be the cause of AIDS. (It was only later that HTLVIII was shown to be none other than Professor Montagnier's LAV.)

The *New Scientist* report, which set off the most bizarre sequence of events in medical history, read as follows: "Researchers at America's National Cancer Institute in Bethesda, Maryland, believe they have finally tracked down the organism that causes Acquired Immuno-Deficiency Syndrome (AIDS). It is a virus that affects particular cells of the immune system and is called Human T cell Leukemia Virus III (HTLVIII)."

In his book *The HIV Myth* (Macmillan, 1989), English journalist Jad Adams described the events that immediately followed the *New Scientist* report:

> "There now occurred one of the strangest tableaux of the entire AIDS story. The Department of Health and Human Services held a press conference in Washington, DC, on April 23 to report on a new virus which had been found by Robert Gallo.
>
> The press conference was held in a small auditorium; too small to hold the reporters and TV

---

[2] The *New Scientist* is not a medical journal. It is a popular weekly magazine on sale to the general public.

crews who attended. Microphones hung round the
lectern like fruit weighing down a tree, and scientists
crowded onto the tiny stage. Secretary of Health
and Human Resources, Margaret Heckler, even
introduced a scientist who wasn't there.

Gallo made a grand entrance, as described by
David Black: 'He approached the podium like the
only kid in the school assembly to have won a
National Merit Scholarship. He was fastidiously
dressed. None of Sonnabend's[3] ratty sweaters and
baggy slacks for him. He wore aviator glasses—a
Hollywood touch—and his hair was rumpled, but
just enough to make it look as if he had recently
emerged from handling a crisis. His manner seemed
to me condescending, as though he were the Keeper
of Secrets obliged to deal with a world of lesser
mortals.' The moral seems to be to make sure David
Black is your friend before you invite him to your
press conference.

Margaret Heckler acknowledged 'other
discoveries . . . in different laboratories—even in
different parts of the world' but the accolade was
reserved for the US: 'Today we add another miracle
to the long honor roll of American medicine and
science.'

Heckler said the discovery of the virus would
allow the development of a vaccine against AIDS
which would be available by 1986. She resigned her
post in 1985 and was sent to Ireland as ambassador.

An honorable exception to the shabby behavior
of the US media in general was the *New York Times*
which, days before the press conference, featured
a story in which credit for the isolation of the virus
went to the Pasteur Institute. Later the *New York
Times* commented on the fierce—and premature—
fight for credit between scientists and bureaucratic
sponsors of research.

[3] Dr Sonnabend—*see* Chapters 7 and 9.

One other event occurred on April 23: a patent was filed in the US on a test kit developed by Gallo. The prestige of coming first in the race to grow the virus was now indistinguishable from the financial gain each institute would receive if they could prove they came first. *The small matter of proving that the virus actually caused the disease remained."*

Conclusion

The small matter of proving that the virus caused the disease *still* remains, and it remains for two very good reasons:

1 There is no valid evidence that the virus causes AIDS.
2 There is an enormous weight of evidence to show that it does not.

So far the HIV theory of AIDS has been sustained in the absence of proof by the very fact it was sponsored and officially launched by the US Federal Government agency, the National Institute of Health. Such credibility was enough for people everywhere to accept the virus theory without question, particularly in view of the fact few doctors know much about viruses anyway, especially "retro"-viruses. And since the official launching of the HIV theory it has been sustained by a constant stream of propaganda from the National Institute of Health's instrumentalities, the Center of Disease Control and the Food and Drug Administration, which contains information relating only to HIV infection rates and so on, completely excluding any of the valuable original research data which on its own invalidates the HIV theory.

The HIV pantomime is nearly over, having had a surprisingly long run. It started in Washington DC, and that's where it will finish, although most of the action has been generated in California. The man who has done most to dispel the myth of HIV and to put some common sense back into medicine is the world's leading virologist,

Professor Peter Duesberg of the University of California, Berkley. Selected in 1987 by the National Institute of Health as one of America's twenty-three most brilliant scientists, Duesberg was awarded the prestigious $500,000 Outstanding Investigator Grant. Great things were expected of him in the war against AIDS, and great things he has indeed achieved—but not (to the dismay of the establishment) quite along the lines they anticipated.

As the world's leading retro-virologist, Professor Duesberg has always insisted emphatically that no retrovirus could possibly be the cause of AIDS. He has over and over again challenged Dr Robert Gallo, the initiator of the HIV hypothesis, or anybody else from the medical establishment, to debate the HIV argument: any time, any place, but there have been no takers. Instead he has had his Outstanding Investigator Grant terminated and his challenges to debate have been ignored or brushed aside as being trivial. But the challenges are not trivial, and sooner or later will have to be answered. In more and more news articles journalists are demanding these answers and coming out in support of Duesberg. Professor Luc Montagnier of the Pasteur Institute in Paris, the very man who discovered HIV in 1983, has stated publicly he no longer believes the virus to be the cause of AIDS. Dr Robert Gallo, the man who dishonestly claimed to first discover HIV and then initiated the HIV hypothesis in 1984, is now back-pedalling on the HIV theory as his credibility dwindles and investigations of fraud threaten the reputation of his entire establishment.

As this book goes to press, a news report from Paris (the *Australian*, 21 April 1992) reads as follows:

Panel Clears HIV Scientist of Plagiarism
by Helen Evans in Paris
An American researcher, Dr Robert Gallo, accused by French scientists of improperly taking credit for discovering the AIDS virus, has been cleared of misconduct by a team of investigators.

The decision by France's Office of Scientific

Integrity came after a two-year investigation into accusations of scientific misconduct by the Gallo team.

Although Dr Gallo was cleared by the report, charges of scientific misconduct were retained against his main collaborator, Mikulas Popovic.

At stake in the battle are royalties from the commercialisation of the diagnostic test for the virus, which are shared equally by France and the United States. It was unclear last night if that arrangement would change.

Scientists at the Pasteur Institute in Paris accuse US researchers of using scientist Dr Luc Montagnier's AIDS virus without giving credit to his French research team, an accusation partially backed up by the report.

The study found US researchers succeeded in isolating samples of the virus before receiving the French sample, but should have given credit to the French for isolating the initial virus.

Dr Gallo and Dr Montagnier are officially considered co-discoverers of the virus under a 1987 agreement between Paris and Washington.

The French Minister of Research, Mr Hubert Curien, said he thought the agreement should be renegotiated.''

From this report it would appear that a two-year investigation has found enough evidence of scientific misconduct to warrant charges against Gallo's closest collaborator Popovic, but at the same time not sufficient evidence to involve Popovic's closest collaborator, Gallo. Does this mean Dr Gallo does not know what is going on in his own inner sanctum? One way or the other he has blown it, because if he doesn't know what is going on under his nose in his own laboratory, what chance has he of knowing what goes on in the microscopic world of cells and viruses?

With due respect to the French Office of Scientific Integrity, it is becoming more and more evident that the

medical management of the AIDS problem has been
nothing less than farcical ever since the HIV theory was
swallowed, hook, line and sinker, by almost everybody in
1984, at the same time reeking in some circles of gross
ineptitude, deceit and greed for money.

Addendum

**A CONVERSATION WITH PETER DUESBERG,
Professor of Virology, University of California, Berkeley**
(from the *California Monthly*, Journal of the University
of California Alumni Association).

"It does not exist on the front pages of newspapers, and
can be found in the scientific literature only after a careful
search, but there is a countermovement in AIDS thinking,
long present and continuing to grow. The
countermovement opposes the standard view that a
retrovirus, Human Immunodeficiency Virus (HIV), is the
cause of Acquired Immune Deficiency Syndrome. The
accepted account of how people with AIDS become ill is
that HIV kills T-cells, the very basis of the immune system;
this allows the introduction of any of 25 diseases into the
defenseless body, which then succumbs.

"This explanation, however, incorporates a number
of paradoxes. First, HIV never infects sufficient numbers
of T-cells to destroy the immune system. Second, according
to this view, disease results from the "AIDS virus" only
after anti-viral immunity has been achieved—that is, only
after antibodies to the virus can be detected. Third, disease
strikes only about ten years after infection (the "latent
period"). Fourth, people with AIDS succumb to different
diseases depending on their risk group (Kaposi's sarcoma
for homosexuals, pneumocystis pneumonia for IV drug
users) or their country of origin (the pneumonia common
in the United States and Europe is not seen among AIDS
sufferers in Africa). Finally, if HIV acted like a conventional
virus, it would by now have spread far beyond its original

points of attack. The virus would be random in the population, as was predicted in 1983, when it was discovered; this, however, has not come to pass.

"The response of the dominant medical groups, private and public, has not been to seek other explanations for AIDS. Instead, billions of dollars have been given to research aimed at resolving the maze of paradoxes surrounding the 'virus-AIDS' hypothesis.

"But many scientists believe that other approaches must be used to explain and therefore deal with AIDS. One of the key figures in this countermovement is Peter Duesberg, a molecular biologist at Berkeley. A member of the National Academy of Science, one of the world's most respected retrovirologists, and a current beneficiary (one of only two on the Cal campus) of an Outstanding Investigator Grant from the National Cancer Institute, the 53-year-old Duesberg has been at Berkeley since 1964.

"Duesberg entered the AIDS debate in 1987, when he wrote *Retroviruses as Carcinogens and Pathogens: Expectations and Reality*, in *Cancer Research*, which closed with an attack on the virus-AIDS hypothesis. In 1988, he debated the issue in the pages of *Science* magazine (*HIV does Not Cause AIDS*). Last year, he wrote *HIV Fails as the Cause of AIDS* in the *Proceedings of the National Academy of Science*.

"He has just completed an article for publication in *Research in Immunology*, *AIDS: Non-infectious deficiencies acquired by drug consumption and other risk factors*, which continues his assault on the virus-AIDS hypothesis and introduces, for the first time, his own proposal, the 'risk-AIDS' hypothesis. With this new hypothesis, he claims to have resolved many of the paradoxes in the standard account. It is the difference between these two accounts which forms the basis for this Q&A.

"Q: I want to explore the differences between the accepted AIDS explanation and the new one you are proposing. What is the standard, 'virus-AIDS', hypothesis?

A: It basically says that AIDS is an infectious, contagious disease, caused by a virus. It holds that the 25 'indicator diseases' of AIDS are all the result of a primary effect of the virus, which is the depletion of T-cells, one of the major components of the immune system.

Q: What are the main diseases, and are any of them new?

A: The major diseases are pneumocystis pneumonia, Kaposi's sarcoma, and dementia. Not one of the 25 is new, although the whole syndrome is often referred to as a 'new disease'—in *Scientific American*, as well as the popular press. But this is clearly not the case. AIDS is not a new disease or a disease at all. What is new is that some of these diseases now occur in a group of people in which they formerly were virtually absent, or at least not observed in the Western, affluent countries. Twenty years ago, we didn't see 20-, 30-, or 40-year-olds with Kaposi's sarcoma, pneumonia, or dementia in the numbers we see now.

Q: And the standard explanation is that we're seeing these diseases in these people now because of the spread of the HIV virus?

A: It's a virus, but a special type of virus in that it's different from many other viruses we know that cause disease in man and animals. It's a retrovirus, and retroviruses in fact are the most benign of viruses: they want to become part of the cell; that's how they survive. Most viruses—the ones that cause polio, flu, measles, mumps, and so forth—kill cells. A retrovirus does not.

Q: But the HIV hypothesis is that it kills immune cells, specifically T-cells.

A: That's one of the many paradoxes of the virus-AIDS hypothesis. Immune deficiency due to a depletion of T-cells is the hallmark of AIDS; yet not more than one in 10,000 T-cells is ever actively infected by HIV. And 'infection' at this rate cannot damage the body.

Q: You're saying that HIV is incapable of killing the cells it's supposed to kill. How do the virus-AIDS thinkers get around this point?

A: The primary technique is to ignore the point. The other approach is to propose hypotheses about the hypothesis.

The hypothesis is that the virus does it. And since the virus doesn't infect T-cells—and my critics agree that more than 99 percent of T-cells are uninfected—they come up with hypotheses about how the virus could possibly kills cells that are not infected. I could count probably a dozen hypotheses that have been put forward. And billions of dollars in research projects are being spent to find out if any of these hypotheses has a chance to succeed.

Q: The January 1990 issue of the *Lancet* carried reports that Kaposi's sarcoma appears in men who are HIV-negative. How does this square with the virus-AIDS hypothesis?

A: It doesn't. You see, Kaposi's was one of the most characteristic AIDS diseases for homosexuals in the early 1980s. When you said Kaposi's, that meant AIDS. What I have asked for some time is 'If HIV is the cause of Kaposi's sarcoma, why are only homosexuals getting it?' They were getting it in the lungs, the face, and the chest—the routes along which amyl nitrite inhalants, or 'poppers', are used. Poppers have been directly correlated with the incidence of Kaposi's sarcoma—the only people in the United States to get Kaposi's were the homosexuals who were using poppers as an aphrodisiac. And as the use of poppers declined—when it was pointed out that this was a dangerous practice—the incidence of Kaposi's sarcoma declined.

I had also wondered why there are Kaposi's sarcoma cases that are free of HIV. How can you get exactly the same disease in the same risk group without HIV? That's usually the kiss of death in an etiology study: if you can get the same disease without the agent, the agent can't be the cause.

So, to answer your question, HIV has nothing to do with Kaposi's sarcoma, as the *Lancet* now agrees, even though this was the original hallmark disease of AIDS.

Q: Then what is the connection between HIV and AIDS?

A: I think that HIV is totally irrelevant as an etiological agent in AIDS. HIV is, by definition, a part of AIDS because AIDS is defined as any of 25 diseases when they occur in the presence of antibody to the virus. But I see no evidence

that it could play any role whatsoever in causing AIDS.
Q: But clearly people do have HIV, or antibodies to HIV, in their blood. What does this mean?
A: You may call it, at least in this country, a surrogate marker for risk behavior. It is very difficult to pick up because the virus is mostly latent; therefore, to pick it up you have to have lots of contacts with other people. And that is essentially the same as saying you're practicing risk behavior.
Q: Sexual promiscuity?
A: Sex is one way. But, as we know from the literature, sex is an extremely inefficient way. On the average, 500 sexual contacts are required to pick up the latent HIV from a partner. That's a lot of contacts.

You could pick it up from a blood transfusion. And you clearly could receive it from your mother—that's how it is naturally transmitted in Africa, perinatally. That's how virtually all retroviruses in animals are transmitted, from mother to offspring. That's why it is found in both sexes and in very high percentages of the population in some countries, like Zaire.
Q: Which means what?
A: Which simply means that in Africa it is an endemic retrovirus, harmless, of which there are many examples in the animal kingdom and even in some humans.
Q: If HIV is harmless, and endemic in parts of Africa, what is causing the deaths there that we are told are due to AIDS?
A: Most of it, I think, is a matter of giving old diseases a new name. I think slim disease, fever, diarrhea—the main AIDS diseases in Africa—have existed there all along.
Q: Caused by what?
A: Malnutrition and parasitic infection, which is far more common there than here. The water is unsterile, the food isn't as clean as it is here, and the nutrition is protein-deficient. A balanced diet would solve most of the health problems in Africa.

Throughout the world, protein malnutrition is the most common cause of disease. The AIDS diseases in fact are the diseases of the poor we had in Europe and the United States a century ago.

We're told that AIDS is a microbial disease, a microbial epidemic. The epidemic exists, but it is not a microbial epidemic. It is a drug epidemic associated with malnutrition.

Q: A drug epidemic?

A: Yes, we are seeing, in the United States, some of the results of the drug culture which has reached epidemic proportions. In particular, psychoactive drugs, which are used by exactly the groups that are said to be at risk for HIV infection.

Q: What are the risk groups?

A: Essentially 90 percent of AIDS cases are in two major risk groups—intravenous drug users and male homosexuals—as they have been since 1981. And I think it should be pointed out that it is not 'male homosexuality' which is the risk—homosexuality is as old as life, and it hasn't become any more dangerous in 1980 than it was in Socrates' and Plato's day.

We are looking at a very small segment of the homosexual population, namely those who are very active because they are aided by psychoactive drugs: cocaine, crack, amphetamines, poppers. And the conventional drugs that compensate for these: Valium, cigarettes, and alcohol. These individuals also get a lot of venereal infections, which require treatment by antibiotics. And with drug addiction often comes protein malnutrition. If you eat junk food and take drugs, you don't make T-cells and B-cells. And if that goes on for eight or ten years, it may become irreversible. And then you're talking about AIDS.

Q: What is your alternative to the virus-AIDS hypothesis?

A: I call it the 'risk-AIDS' hypothesis. It proposed that non-infectious agents, such as psychoactive drugs, over-medication with antibiotics, and now, above all, AZT, are causing immune deficiencies and other deficiencies that are now called AIDS.

Q: Let's talk about AZT, the only federally approved treatment for AIDS. What is it?

A: AZT is simply an analogue of one of the four building blocks of DNA. It's essentially chemotherapy—it was developed to treat leukemia—designed to kill fast-growing cells. In the case of AIDS, it's aimed particularly at lymphocytes, the immune system. It kills cells. That's the one thing we can say for sure about it.

Q: What is the rationale for killing cells as part of AIDS therapy?

A: Those who sanction AZT say that they don't want to kill cells, they want to interfere with the replication of the virus. Retroviruses make DNA; AZT inhibits DNA synthesis. Everything that is in the process of making DNA will be killed by AZT.

Q: Won't it kill the person who takes it?

A: It will kill the person. AZT proponents say, 'This is the price you pay for killing the virus.' And they think the benefits are worth that cost.

Q: But government reports have said that AZT prolongs AIDS patients' lives.

A: I have never seen any such study. That was science by press release. No studies have ever been published to back up those claims. I have asked people in the field, I have written to the *New York Times* and other papers which repeated the government claims, and I have never gotten an answer. I don't know what to call this type of propaganda.

Q: What do you think of treating AIDS patients with AZT?

A: I think there is no rational basis for treating any AIDS patient with AZT. The first reason is that we have no proof that HIV is the cause of AIDS. Second, even if we had such proof, the number of infected cells which would be the rational targets for AZT therapy—the sole justification for the therapy, to kill HIV-infected cells—is so incredibly low that the toxicity index will be irresponsibly high. The net result is an incredible attack on the immune system. Which is exactly why you have AIDS, according to the standard definition. So with AZT you'll take out the little bit of the immune system that is left.

Thus, in my opinion, AZT treatment is totally

irresponsible. I would be more forgiving if we were talking about a drug like aspirin, which we don't totally understand and which might have some miraculous side effect. But AZT is not one of those drugs. AZT is a drug whose mechanism is embarrassingly clear. There is no possible way you could see a beneficial side effect of a chain terminator of DNA synthesis. I don't see how this could be justified. At all.

Q: If what you say is true, how can people stand by and let this happen?

A: I have asked myself this question many times. The only answer I can come up with is that they have made this look so confusing and complex that many people say, 'I don't know enough to judge this.' In fact, I think that the majority of people who believe in the virus-AIDS hypothesis are totally unaware that the virus is completely latent at the time you get AIDS and infects very, very few cells. People don't check the details of popular dogma or consensus views. I know that many people in the field who have been asked to respond to my scientific papers on the subject say they haven't had the time to read them. Many have said straight out that they won't read them. 'Duesberg's off the wall.' Or: 'He's from Berkeley.'

Another part of it is that most people, even scientists, take their information from the newspapers. Science is really now a popularity contest, made by newspapers. You hype something in the press, and people take it from there. They do not advertise the fact that HIV infects only one in 10,000 cells. If people are really pushed on this point, they come up with a dozen hypotheses that could—but so far don't—explain it.

Finally, I think another reason is that many AIDS scientists have significant commercial interests in companies that are tied to the HIV-AIDS hypothesis. If you open up the AZT question, then the viral cause of AIDS must come up. And that would raise a lot of flack.

Q: Let's return to your alternative to the virus-AIDS hypothesis. How will the 'risk-AIDS' hypothesis help?

A: My alternative, I believe, will explain in a rational way virtually everything that is paradoxical in the virus-AIDS hypothesis—25 diseases in the presence of antibodies to a retrovirus which I consider harmless because it is always idle.

My hypothesis postulates that most of the AIDS diseases in the United States and Europe are a direct consequence of the consumption of psychoactive drugs. Thirty percent of AIDS cases in this country are confirmed IV-drug users. We don't need any further explanation for those. And the others we have briefly discussed: the homosexuals who are at risk. for AIDS use batteries of drugs—as aphrodisiacs, to get high, or for medical purposes. The worst of them now, of course, is AZT.

The risk-AIDS hypothesis would help explain why different groups get different diseases. As I said before, generally speaking the homosexuals in this country are the only ones to get Kaposi's sarcoma and they are the only ones who use poppers. Heroin and cocaine addicts get pneumonia. In Africa, they get slim disease and fever and diarrhea because of straight malnutrition and all the local infections there; they don't get pneumonia, even though they carry the same pneumocystis in their lungs that people in the rest of the world do. So, all of these groups are at risk, not because of HIV but because of the damage done to their bodies, directly or indirectly; by drugs and malnutrition.

My alternative, then, would explain why AIDS remains exclusively restricted to the major risk groups and is not random in the population, as an infectious disease would be. It would explain why it takes, on the average, ten years after infection to develop symptoms—ten years is merely an expression of the long and unpredictable time it takes to reach a threshold for pathogenicity when you use toxic drugs or have a toxic lifestyle.

Q: What is the 'toxic lifestyle' of a hemophiliac?
A: Being a hemophiliac puts one at risk for a number of diseases. One element is the immunosuppressive function of blood substances—whether it is Factor VIII for hemophiliacs or blood transfusions in general. Both of these

are known, classical conditions that repress the immune system. Again, it's individually very different. Some people accept blood products better than others.

And of course the additional risk is that, despite all current precautions, there are accidental infections that accompany blood products: hepatitis, cytomegalo infection, Epstein–Barr infection, and other infections through transfusions. That's unfortunately not uncommon.

Q: What about press reports of a year or two ago about the 55-year-old Marin woman who died of AIDS five years after receiving a blood transfusion?

A: That is what is called an anecdotal study; it's worthless for science. You need a controlled study to identify the cause of a disease in a person who picked up a presumably causative virus—or antibody to a virus—five years earlier. You would need a hundred 55-year-old women from Marin County who got the same disease she did—what was it, pneumonia?—and are antibody positive. And you would need to compare them to a hundred similar 55-year-old women without antibody to the virus. If only the hundred antibody-positive women became sick, and the only variable were the virus, then you could say the virus could have done it.

I want to emphasize that such a controlled study has never been done. Not a single one. I have asked for such studies. I have suggested them. A good one would be to match hemophiliacs with and without antibody to the virus, follow them for a year or more, and then ask: How are the ones with antibody doing compared to those without antibody? If you found pneumonia, hepatitis, cytomegalovirus, and all the other infections that are typical of hemophilia only in the ones with antibody to the virus, then you'd have some evidence.

Q: What do you expect would be found from such a controlled study?

A: The incidence of AIDS diseases in HIV-positives and HIV-negatives would be exactly the same.

If you think a virus is the cause of AIDS, do a control without it. To do a control is the first thing you teach undergraduates. But it hasn't been done. The epidemiology of AIDS is a pile of anecdotal stories, selected to fit the virus-AIDS hypothesis.

Q: You are saying that AIDS is not an infectious disease?

A: Yes. It doesn't fit anything we know about infectious diseases. It stays in risk groups; it takes ten years from so-called infection to symptoms. Microbes are not that picky—to limit themselves to very special risk groups. There is no microbe that takes ten years to cause disease. Within a couple of weeks or months, either you reject the microbe or the microbe eats you up.

I think you can ask one question after another that was not answered by the virus-AIDS hypothesis and answer it with the risk-AIDS hypothesis. It explains, for example, why a vaccine would never work. Because antibodies to the virus are said to be the *precondition* for AIDS under the standard definition. An absolute paradox. It would be the first and only virus in the universe that causes 25 different diseases *only after anti-viral immunity*! But this paradox could readily be reconciled with the hypothesis of risk- or drug-induced diseases. According to this hypothesis, the roughly ten years HIV is said to take to cause disease—the so-called latent period—would depend on how often you use drugs, what drugs you use, where you inject them, and how sensitive your body is to them. Thresholds would be largely different for different people, and the outcomes would therefore be largely different— as they are in AIDS cases.

Q: You think the war on AIDS should, instead, be the war on drugs?

A: Yes, I think so. But that is not my field. I am just trying to find a consistent alternative, trying to find an explanation. And I think the only thing new in the past 15 years in the Western world is the increased use of drugs.

Q: What about AIDS in babies in this country?

A: An AIDS baby is one who is (a) sick and (b) has antibody to the virus. Now, 95 percent of AIDS babies are born to mothers who are drug-addicted or prostitutes. That's 95 percent of the cases. You don't hear of AIDS babies in

Orinda or Lafayette. Never. You're talking about children who have picked up the virus from their mothers. And the babies are sick and die because the mother, say, was taking cocaine when she should have had a steak or a glass of milk, at the time the baby's lung was being formed or the brain was being developed—this is an extremely sensitive time for the baby, the early stages of development. If it doesn't get proteins at this time, it will be retarded or defective; it can't catch up.

Q: What difference does it make which hypothesis you use—virus-AIDS or risk-AIDS? People are still dying.

A: Well, it makes a difference if you want to develop a public-health policy that is successful. The one we have now, based on the virus-AIDS hypothesis, is a total failure. Its predictions are wrong: AIDS hasn't spread into the heterosexual population. Current policy hasn't cured anyone, despite the billions of dollars spent. And it now is using AZT, which will kill more and more people. These are the accomplishments of the virus-AIDS hypothesis translated into public-health policy.

So if you want to have a better showing in terms of public-health benefits, you first have to know what the cause is and then take appropriate action. But you'll never get a good public-health policy based on poor science. And that's what we have now.

A public-health policy based on the risk-AIDS hypothesis would immediately break away from the central HIV definition of the syndrome and instead would classify the 25 diseases according to the risks that may generate them—poppers for Kaposi's, heroin for pneumonia—and would treat each one accordingly. You wouldn't give all of these people AZT regardless of whether they are suffering from diarrhea or dementia or Kaposi's sarcoma or pneumonia—which is what we're doing now.

Q: If a person is HIV-positive but does not take drugs, eats a balanced diet, and gets good exercise and rest, what is his prognosis?

A: Exactly the same as for an HIV-negative person. Exactly the same. The fact that one or two million Americans are antibody positive, and no more than 20,000 a year, or 1.5 percent, develop one of these 25 diseases is already an indication that being antibody-positive can't be a big risk factor by itself. And these one or two million Americans include, of course, most of those who have used lots of drugs.

Q: Although you're not talking about sexual practices, the fact that you are talking about drug use recalls the earlier versions of 'lifestyle' as the cause of AIDS.

A: Non-infectious agents seem to be called lifestyle, and that implies responsibility or blame. If the cause is a virus, no one can help it. I talked to an AIDS group recently, and they were sensitive to the 'risk-AIDS' hypothesis. They said, 'You're saying we are doing bad things, bringing this on ourselves.'

Q: What was your response?

A: I said, 'I'm a scientist, not a politician or a priest. My only interest is to find a solution for AIDS. Or at least an explanation. Once you have an explanation that makes sense, then you can debate public health policies.'

Q: You have been both ignored and vilified since you came out against HIV as the cause of AIDS. What do you see as you look ahead?

A: I'm a little more optimistic than I was a year or two ago. I think my best ally is the truth. The virus hypothesis simply doesn't make any sense. It is so poorly framed, and like all poorly framed hypotheses, it doesn't generate any benefits. It has yet to save the first patient. And we are about to kill off, intoxicate, 50,000 people with AZT. That's the number now taking AZT. And that's the same number of people we lost in Vietnam.

This is now 1990, by which time AIDS was supposed to have killed off the Haitians and to have moved into the heterosexual population because it was a sexually transmitted disease. But we don't hear anything any more—in the press or in the scientific literature—about Haitians. And the primary risk groups, drug users and homosexuals, have remained the same as they were at the beginning. All of these paradoxes had to be incorporated into the virus-

AIDS hypothesis: This virus is so special and so smart that it causes a disease in homosexuals it wouldn't cause in drug addicts, causes different diseases in Africa than in Europe, and it waits ten years to do so.

I think people will soon wake up and ask, 'Why are we spending a billion dollars a year on a hypothesis that has yet to save a single life.' "

Statement by Robert S. Roote-Bernstein, Associate Professor of Physiology, Michigan State University, East Lansing, MI (as appeared in *Policy Review*, Fall 1990).
Professor Roote-Bernstein is, like Professor Duesberg, a member of a select group of twenty-three chosen by the National Cancer Institute as the most brilliant scientists in America, and as such is the recipient of the prestigious Outstanding Investigator Grant.

"Lest readers of Duesberg and Ellison's article claiming that HIV is not the cause of AIDS think that the authors are lone wolves crying in the wilderness, let me add my voice to the growing chorus. While I am not convinced that HIV is irrelevant to understanding AIDS—after all it is highly correlated with the syndrome—I am not convinced that it is any more important than other immunosuppressive agents associated with AIDS. On the contrary, I believe existing evidence demonstrates that HIV is neither necessary nor sufficient to cause AIDS.

"First, data linking HIV to AIDS are nowhere near as good as the public are led to believe. Reference to the Centers for Disease Control's own data reveals that 5 percent of AIDS patients tested for HIV never display signs of infection, and that less than 50 percent of AIDS patients have been tested for HIV.

"Recently, cases of homosexual men with AIDS and without HIV infections have been verified. In response, HIV proponents are lobbying for a change in the definition of AIDS to exclude HIV-free cases. These people do not, apparently, understand two things: 1) that defining AIDS by HIV and simultaneously demonstrating that HIV causes

AIDS is tautological, and therefore bankrupt, reasoning; and 2) that altering the definition of AIDS does not alter the fact that HIV-free people can and do develop the same set of opportunistic infections as those who are HIV-infected. Whether these HIV-free cases are listed as AIDS patients or not, they are still medical patients whose syndrome is in need of explanation. Logically, HIV is not, therefore, necessary to cause the development of these symptoms, and other causes of what we now call AIDS must exist.

Other Agents

"My own research, which was published this summer in *Perspectives in Biology and Medicine*, suggests what these other causes of acquired immunosuppression may be. Briefly summarized, all of the following agents had been demonstrated to be immunosuppressive prior to the discovery of HIV, and all are highly associated with one or more AIDS risk groups: immunological response to semen following anal intercourse; the use of recreational drugs such as the nitrites ('poppers' and 'snappers'); chronic antibiotic use (often associated with promiscuity); opiate drugs; multiple transfusions; anesthetics; malnutrition (whether caused by 'gay bowel syndrome', drug use, poverty, or anorexia nervosa); multiple, concurrent infections by diverse microbes; and infection by specific viruses such as cytomegalovirus, Epstein–Barr virus, and hepatitis-B virus (all of which are as highly associated with AIDS as is HIV).

"Several of these agents, including cytomegalovirus, hepatitis-B virus, opiate drugs, and repeated blood transfusions, are known to cause the same sort of T-cell abnormalities that are found in AIDS, and which are usually attributed (perhaps inaccurately) to HIV infection. The other agents cause a wider spectrum of immunosuppressive responses, and probably explain why more than simply T-cells are non-functional in AIDS patients. Every AIDS patient has several of these immunosuppressive agents at work in his or her system in addition to, and sometimes in the absence of, HIV. We cannot, therefore, logically conclude that HIV is the sole or even the main cause of immunosuppression in AIDS.

19th-Century AIDS

"Now, if the so-called life-style theory of AIDS is correct, one important implication is that AIDS should not be a new syndrome. It is not. I am one of only a handful of scientists who have bothered to search intensively through the back issues of medical journals for odd cases that match the CDC surveillance definition of AIDS. So far I have found hundreds of such cases, extending back to 1872 (the date when the first opportunistic disease associated with AIDS was identified). I have also scoured the medical literature for data relevant to changes in life-style risks associated with immunosuppression. What I have found is very provocative.

"Whereas the Kinsey report of 1948 indicates that the average homosexual man had a sexual encounter no more frequently than once a month, by 1980, the advent of gay bars and bath houses had increased this average to dozens per month. Gay AIDS patients have often had thousands of sexual partners. Medical reports of complications arising from AIDS-associated high-risk activities such as anal intercourse and fisting are first mentioned in the medical literature only at the beginning of the 1970s, and become increasingly frequent thereafter. From 1960 to 1980, the rates of syphilis triple, gonorrhoea quadruple, and diseases related to 'gay bowel syndrome' quadruple. These increases were found only among gay men, but not among heterosexual men or women.

"From 1960 to 1980, hepatitis-B cases rose 10-fold, in part due to sexual transmission in gay men, and in part to IV drug abuse. Arrests on opiate-related drug charges rose nearly 20-fold during the same period. There is, then, no doubt that AIDS was preceded by medically evident changes in life-style among those groups at highest risk for AIDS, and these changes are such that not only HIV, but the entire spectrum of immunosuppressive agents mentioned above became increasingly prevalent in these groups.

"These data indicate to me that HIV is not sufficient to explain the manifestation of AIDS or its recent appearance. Many other factors are also at work. It is a tremendous mistake to base our policy decisions concerning AIDS on an exclusive HIV basis. Far from undermining current drug prevention and safe sex programs, the recognition of non-HIV immunosuppressive factors in AIDS suggests that these programs are failing because they are *too narrow*. AIDS will only be understood when we begin to explore the ways in which anal sex, infections, drugs, blood products, anesthetics, antibiotics, and malnutrition interact. At present, we know almost nothing about such interactions. Since increasing evidence from the laboratories of the discoverers of HIV indicates that HIV needs immunosuppressive co-factors to be active, such studies are clearly needed. In the meantime, those who wish to avoid contracting AIDS should avoid all potential causes of immunosuppression, not just HIV. And those who are HIV-positive but not ill may find that if they, too, avoid the lengthy list of immunosuppressive co-factors, they too will stay healthy."

CHAPTER 9

The Drug Business

The disgrace of medicine has been that colossal system of self-deception, in obedience to which mines have been emptied of their cankering minerals, the entrails of animals taken for their impurities, the poison bag of reptiles drained for their venom, and all the inconceivable absurdities thus obtained thrust down the throats of human beings suffering simply of some want of organization, nourishment or vital stimulation.

If all the drugs were cast into the sea, it would be so much better for man, and so much the worse for the fishes.

Oliver Wendell Holmes (1809–94)

When people think about the appalling effects of drugs in the world there comes to mind pictures of heavily armed drug barons in jungle hideaways, drug pick-ups from darkened boats offshore and from secret airstrips, of evil mafia characters, drug pushers and emaciated addicts. We think of young people lying dead in untidy rooms or in back alleys.

That alcohol and cigarettes, albeit in a slower way, wreck more lives and physically destroy far more people than illegal drugs does not arouse all that much concern because they have long been an established part of our culture, considered by many to be quite an essential part. The people who control the liquor and tobacco industries and who push their products in lavish advertising sprees would have to be as morally corrupt as any jungle drug baron, but instead of being hounded by the law they are looked upon, often in admiration, as dynamic and successful businessmen.

Be that as it may, that's what we've got, and everybody knows it. But what everybody does not know is that there is a more insidious and widespread drug danger to humanity than all the others put together, and that is the ever-increasing consumption of pharmaceutical products which, in terms of money, corruption and danger, makes the operation of jungle drug barons look like chickenfeed. The pharmaceutical companies don't just target impressionable teenagers for their next crop of addicts; they target everybody, young and old.

Almost everyone at some time or another takes medicine either bought over the counter or prescribed by their doctor, without for one second querying whether it may be anything other than good for them. They are entitled to feel that way because they trust their doctor and respect his vast knowledge. If only they knew just how little he really knew!

Regardless of whatever effect is conveyed by medicine, it is a fact that any chemical substance—other than those in natural nutrients—that enters the bloodstream is sensed by the body as a poison to be neutralized and eliminated as quickly as possible, and it is the job of the liver, kidneys, immune system and other vital organs to achieve this. Because most medicines are not virulent poisons, they can be neutralized and eliminated without too much difficulty, and if adverse effects are experienced they are defined medically to be only "side effects"—a term that sounds better than poisoning. However, with or without side effects the body's systems—no doubt already overburdened with other toxins to start with—has been put under even greater strain, and it is no wonder that after many years of drug-treated chronic illness, one or another of the vital organs breaks down and death of the patient ensues. The patient's death is reported in the local news as having occurred after a long illness—which is true—but it would be more accurate to say that the death was consequential to a long process of poisoning the patient could no longer endure.

Iatrogenic disease[1] has always been known to be a major cause of death, and if allowance is made for the undetected and unrecorded cases it would be reasonable, in the light of current knowledge, to assume iatrogenic disease to be one of the very main causes of death. The reason why a doctor can unknowingly poison a patient to death is that even if he knows there will be side effects, he has no option if he is to please his patient other than to prescribe the "approved" medicine, and he is equipped with little knowledge as to the effects of long-term usage.

To illustrate the fact that vast numbers of sick people are killed by what is called "complications" arising from medical treatment are the occasions in fairly recent years when death rates have fallen dramatically following situations when doctors have gone on strike. In 1973 doctors in Israel went on strike and reduced their daily patient services from 65,000 to only 7000. The strike lasted a month, and during that time the death rate, according to the Jerusalem Burial Society, dropped fifty per cent. In 1976 in Bogota, Columbia, doctors refused to treat all except emergency cases for a period of fifty-two days, and in that time the death rate fell thirty-five per cent. Also in 1976, a slowdown by doctors in Los Angeles resulted in a fall of eighteen per cent in deaths. Too bad for some that it was only a slowdown!

The medical industry of today has become the subsidiary of the pharmaceutical industry, now the wealthiest industry in the world. Doctors of all ranks are today puppets controlled by financial strings. The pharmaceutical companies make such astronomical profits from their position of monopoly that all they have to do to maintain that position is to devote as much money as

---

[1] Iatrogenic means caused by medical treatment. According to a report from the World Health Organization, one in every four hospital deaths is the result of medical drugs—from *The Healing Mind* by Dr Irving Oyle, 1975.

necessary in influencing the right people—which is all of us. The pharmaceutical companies provide or control most of the money for medical research (providing the research meets their approval); they provide large sums to the various medical journals in which they advertise lavishly; they fund lavish holidays for doctors disguised as medical conferences; and they hand out to doctors all sorts of lavish gifts.

A Sydney newspaper recently disclosed some of the methods by which doctors are encouraged by drug companies to prescribe their products. The companies make gifts of computers, briefcases, golf balls, calculators, hotel dinners, conferences at exotic resorts, calenders, beepers, and other give-aways. The companies devoted fifteen per cent of their total sales income to promoting their products, and this amounted to an average of $10,000 for every general medical practitioner in the country.

The drug companies don't have to influence doctors to prescribe drugs—they are already trained to do this; the companies' main concern is that the doctor prescribes the right ones, ie, the ones which are most profitable. So to influence a doctor's decision in this regard the companies have what they call "detail men" (salesmen) who call in on doctors regularly and bring them up-to-date with the new lines available, and it is upon this sort of "know-how" that you, the patient, must depend for relief from your next twinge of arthritis or whatever.

This is the modern practice of medicine, and when organs within the body pack up and fail, scientific medicine steps in and conducts a transplant for you—if you have the money. Such is the system proudly called "health care" by politicians, "scientific medicine" by the chemists and surgeons, and "sound business" by the pharmaceutical companies.

To complete their stranglehold on the medical profession the drug companies maintain a powerful influence within the upper echelons of health and drug administration agencies, which influence is reflected in the agencies' uncompromising opposition of natural health practitioners and anyone else who disagrees with the official allopathic[2] line. It cannot be coincidental that upon retirement, many of the former heads of government agencies find themselves in highly paid jobs in the hierarchies of the drug companies.

Thus is explained the banning of laetrile, the herbal extract demonstrated in the US Food and Drug Administration's own tests to be helpful in the treatment of cancer, and the outlawing of any cancer therapy that does not conform to official medical guidelines, such as therapies based on herbs, vitamins, diet and so on. The thalidomide scandal of the 1960s is a good example of the ethics of the drug trade, and to read the book *Thalidomide and the Power of the Drug Companies* would chill even Jack the Ripper to the bone. Even when thalidomide was publicly exposed as the cause of the dreadful infant deformities happening at the time, the Distillers Company of Germany continued to market the drug in countries where it had not been banned. In the USA the Food and Drug Administration (FDA) was prepared to okay the drug in the face of warnings from one of its own doctors, a lady, and it was only because of this lady's stubborn insistence that thalidomide was not unleashed on the pregnant women of America. How many adult Americans today can thank this courageous woman for their intact bodies will always be unknown, but they certainly don't owe any thanks to the top brass of the FDA.

Today we are witnessing yet another scandal, this time involving the marketing of a dangerous drug by the Burroughs Wellcome Company. This is the drug AZT, which until recently was the only drug approved for the treatment of AIDS, thus giving Burroughs Wellcome a multibillion dollar monopoly in the AIDS industry. The drug was FDA approved without the proper clinical trials, just as on pure supposition HIV was designated the approved cause of AIDS. To make the deal a real push-over for Burroughs Wellcome, they had to make no promises

---

[2] Allopathy is the practise of medicine in which drugs are used to alleviate pain and other symptoms.

or guarantees. All that is claimed for AZT is that it inhibits the spread of HIV in the body, and that—despite the admitted fact that it is poisonous and highly immunosuppressive—it extends the life expectancy of people with AIDS. This claim is still being made despite the fact AZT has been shown to be distinctly of no advantage at all, the claim being sustained by the fact that deaths among HIV-positive people have not been as numerous as predicted. The true position is that HIV-positive people have not perished as predicted because HIV is not the cause of AIDS at all, whereas the prediction was made on the assumption that it was. The tragedy now being enacted is that many reasonably healthy people, merely on the basis of them having HIV antibodies in their blood, are being transformed into sick people by AZT and the tortured thinking that accompanies the belief in HIV. And when AZT destroys their immune system HIV will, of course, get the official blame. As time elapses the fearful consequences of AZT become more apparent; in August 1991 the US National Institute of Health (NIH) revealed that nearly half of AZT patients eventually develop aggressive cancer.

For Burroughs Wellcome to continue with their AZT financial bonanza, it is vitally important for the HIV illusion to be sustained, and they are doing everything they can to sustain it. In 1983 Dr Joseph Sonnabend of New York (*see* previous chapter) started a journal called *AIDS Research* to act as a forum for basic research and general information on AIDS. When the HIV theory was announced in 1984 the journal maintained its impartial stance, including in its contents discussion both for and against the theory. *AIDS Research* was still an independent journal in 1986, with twenty-one people on the editorial board. Then the Burroughs Wellcome company began to fund the journal and shortly afterwards took over control. It is more than significant that Burroughs Wellcome changed the name of the journal to *AIDS Research and Human Retroviruses*, and in its first edition for 1987 the journal contained nine articles, seven of them about HIV and two about other retro-viruses. The editorial board now numbered fifty, of which only two were original members, Dr Sonnabend not being one of them.

AIDS Research was a good name for Dr Sonnabend's journal; why encumber the name by adding "and Retroviruses" to it? Why is it now common in medical literature to refer to AIDS as "HIV disease"? Is it meant to somehow reinforce the belief in HIV and to sustain a theory too weak to stand inspection?

By their control of research funds, upon which the careers of many influential research doctors depend, the drug companies can control what is discovered and what is not, and they are not interested in discoveries that don't lead to selling drugs. Researchers whose work shows no "promise" in this regard soon find themselves short of research funds, and this is why so little progress has been achieved in the "war against cancer" and why no progress at all has been achieved in the "war against AIDS".

The key to winning the war against AIDS is the same key that is needed to win the war against cancer. What has to be overcome is not a germ or a virus, but vested interests and mental blocks which keep research pointing in the wrong direction. The etiology of cancer was obvious to many doctors one hundred years ago but never saw much light of day until clearly explained by four of the world's greatest cancer researchers about forty years ago (*see* Chapter 11). One of them, Dr Otto Warburg, was a double Nobel Prize winner, but his findings did not interest the world of medicine which needs disease to exist and whose interest is only in finding "cures" which can be sold for money. However, the war against AIDS will not be so prolonged because the factors involved are not as obscure as with cancer, and when the HIV pantomime is over and the already known factors are properly assessed, the true etiology of AIDS will be obvious to everybody . . . but only after a lot of people have been killed by AZT and a lot of money made by Burroughs Wellcome.

AZT: The AIDS Drug

AZT, it is admitted by its manufacturers, Burroughs Wellcome, is toxic and suppressive to the immune system. It sounds absurd that something of a toxic and immunosuppressive nature could help someone who is already terribly immuno-compromised, but the theory is that by the drug's effect of inhibiting the action of HIV there is achieved a net gain, so enabling the AIDS patient—supposedly already doomed—to live a little longer.

Now, if HIV was indeed the cause of AIDS, and if indeed AZT worked in the way intended, there would indeed be a case for its use, but leaving the HIV argument right out of it, tests have shown AZT to be at best useless and at worst harmful. On 13–14 February 1991, in Washington DC, a special meeting was held of the Anti-viral Drugs Committee of the Food and Drug Administration (FDA) to discuss the validity of AZT use. The first thing that was agreed upon was that the P24 antigen test, upon which AZT effectiveness was assessed, was useless and meaningless, which of course meant that the grounds upon which AZT was approved in the first place were spurious. The main focus of the meeting was the Veterans Administration Co-operative Study 298, the preliminary findings of which were presented by Dr John Hamilton MD. The study was of 338 HIV-positive individuals with AIDS, divided into two groups, both groups given AZT but in different dosage. Dr Hamilton reported that no benefit for either treatment group was detected for survival or the combined chemical end points of AIDS and death. He said that early AZT resulted in transitory benefits in whites, and neutral or harmful effects in black and Hispanic patients. *No mention was made of the high risk of cancer for those taking the drug.*

The very next day the shares of the Burroughs Wellcome parent company fell[3] by ten per cent, but

---

[3] The author wonders how much further the shares would have fallen if the 50:50 chance of cancer had been mentioned.

Burroughs Wellcome responded quickly the same day with a letter to physicians which they drafted in such a way to indicate the Washington meeting had re-affirmed the previous support for AZT, which was not the case at all. But not to incriminate themselves, they put the onus on the FDA by including a copy of the FDA *Talk Paper* on the subject. Reporter John Lauritsen described the FDA paper thus:

> "The FDA *Talk Paper* dated 14 Feb, 1991, reads as though it had been drafted by Burroughs Wellcome. A more false and distorted version of the meeting could hardly be imagined. The first sentence claims that the committee 're-affirmed the drug's usefulness in treating individuals who are at less advanced stages of infection with the AIDS Virus.' Then the *Talk Paper* goes on to summarize the VA study in such a way as to obliterate the most important finding: that AZT conferred no benefit in terms of survival."

This is how the FDA *Talk Paper* was worded:

> "One study presented to the committee was conducted by the Veterans' Administration. Preliminary results from this study, in general, confirmed that earlier use of zidovudine was beneficial in delaying the onset of AIDS. However, the study when analyzed by various demographic factors also indicated that zidovudine's effects might vary significantly among different patient groups. For unknown reasons, among the African–American and Hispanic patients in the study, those who received zidovudine at a later stage of their infection may have fared better than those who received earlier treatment with the drug. The results regarding the outcome of African–American and Hispanic patients were not conclusive however, and thus no definite changes in practise were deemed appropriate by the Committee."

Reporter Lauritsen concluded: "It should be clear that Burroughs Wellcome is a thoroughly unscrupulous company, and the collusion between the FDA and Burroughs Wellcome is as strong as ever."

The text of John Lauritsen's address to the FDA Committee meeting on 14 February 1991 was as follows:

"I'm John Lauritsen. I'm here as a working journalist, and also as an AIDS Dissident, so my comments will be against the grain. In the United States, AIDS dissidents are not sent to Siberia, the way that dissidents were in the Soviet Union when they disagreed with the tenets of Lysenkoism. However, we are punished. Two physicians who questioned the HIV–AIDS hypothesis had their practices destroyed, and were driven to the edge of bankruptcy. Molecular biologist Peter Duesberg, an outstanding scientist, had a grant cancelled. And I've taken my share of abuse. All this was for questioning what is probably a false hypothesis.

For two decades, I've made my living analyzing statistical data. Before analyzing data, there are two things one needs to know. Number one, are the data good? And number two, are the premises correct—is the study design good? I maintain with regard to AZT that much of the data are bad, and in some cases manifestly fraudulent. And secondly, that most of the AZT research is based on a false hypothesis—the hypothesis that a retrovirus, tendentiously named the Human Immuno-deficiency Virus (HIV) is the cause of AIDS.

I am the author of a book, which has become an underground best seller. It is called *Poison By Prescription: The AZT Story*. It gives quite a different viewpoint from what you have heard here. In this book I come to three main conclusions. Number one: AZT is highly toxic. Number two: AZT was approved for marketing on the basis of research which was not just bad and sloppy and so on, but was overtly, manifestly fraudulent. And three, there is really no scientifically credible evidence that AZT has any benefits.

With regard to toxicity, I would point out that the issue of cancer has been swept under the rug. I didn't hear cancer mentioned once at this meeting. And yet four different lines of proof, of reasoning, indicate that AZT will cause cancer in the long run. First, there are the biochemical properties of the drug itself. Peter Duesberg has pointed out that when a nucleoside analogue is incorporated into a cell, there are only two possible outcomes. Either the cell dies, or, if the cell is lucky, it mutates and the patient gets cancer. Second, there is the Cell Transformation Assay, which was performed several years ago. The results of this test indicated that AZT was highly positive, and therefore should be presumed to be a potential carcinogen. Third, there are the rodent carcinogenicity studies, which found that AZT causes cancer in animals, and therefore probably will in humans as well. And fourth is the correlation, which is becoming ever more clear, between AZT therapy and cancer of the lymph system. The issue of cancer must be taken into consideration when recommending a drug for long-term use.

With regard to the charge of fraud, which I realize is quite serious, I would point out that the Phase II AZT trials occurred when Frank Young was FDA Commissioner. Consumer advocates, such as Sidney Wolfe, charged that Young's reign was one of lawlessness, in terms of collusion between industry and government. Young had to resign, under the shadow of the generic drugs scandal. Illegal collusion between the FDA and drug companies is nothing new. There have been a number of exposès on this topic—by Morton Mintz, by a Ralph Nader study group, and others. Collusion is really business as usual.

With regard to the conflict-of-interest issue, I notice that some of the speakers are identified on the program as Burroughs Wellcome scientists. That's fine, you know that's like truth in advertising or labelling. One is alerted that these people may be giving sales pitches rather than objective presentations of data. However, other people like Margaret Fischl, are not identified as being in the Burroughs Wellcome camp. And yet remuneration, in whatever form it takes, direct or indirect, including grants to institutions, should be taken into account and recognized.

On the question of markers, which was the topic yesterday, I have been writing for some time that the P-24 antigen test is no good. Harvey Bialy, in a forceful editorial in *BioTechnology* several years ago, pointed out that the P-24 antigen test was no good, and that the results from it, which appeared in medical journals, were absurd. It is good to see it recognized now, finally, that the test is useless. However, one should realize that for several years the P-24 antigen test was used to claim benefits for AZT. One can't just forget that. Furthermore, it is more than likely that the P-24 antigen test doesn't mean much for the simple reason that HIV is not the cause of AIDS.

With regard to the CD4 test—it was clear from yesterday's talks that the CD4 test isn't really all that good. However, this is the test that is the basis for giving AZT to people who are objectively healthy. And you are the committee that made the recommendations—to give AZT routinely to people with HIV antibodies, whose CD4 counts fall below 500. I maintain that we are confronted with nothing less than pharmacogenic manslaughter at this point—125,000 people, more or less, are now undergoing AZT therapy. Many of these are objectively healthy people, who ought to live for another 20, 30, or 40 years. I don't think that they

will. I think that they will die of AZT poisoning.
And I think this committee must realize that it has
responsibility. In fact, if I am correct, and we will
know in a few years, this committee has blood on
its hands. If some of you have consciences, and are
not beholden to particular industrial interests, then
you should do what you can, now, to stop this
genocide.

I know that some people refuse to believe in
the possibility of genocide. But genocide has
occurred at other times and in other places, and
it is happening here and now.

There have been many other drug scandals.
Take thalidomide, when the head of the FDA did
everything he could to prevent Frances Kelsey from
doing her job. It was one single independent
woman, a maverick, who prevented thalidomide
from entering the United States. If Frances Kelsey
had not stood up to her superiors, if the FDA had
done business as usual, then thalidomide would
have been marketed in the United States, with the
consequences being thousands of monstrously
deformed infants. And I submit to you that the
thalidomide scandal was utterly trivial—it didn't
amount to a hill of beans—compared to the AZT
scandal that is happening now.

I know some of these people on AZT. You
know, it's not real to think of 125,000 people. But
I know three, or four, or five of the nicest people
I could . . . I could describe. Young, intelligent
people, who ought to live for a long time. And
they will not. They have been persuaded through
lies to take a drug which will surely terminate their
lives long before their time.

Please do your job. Find out the real facts.
Don't believe everything you hear at these meetings,
or that you read in medical journals, about the
alleged benefits of AZT. It is elementary that when
researchers have committed fraud in the past, as

was certainly the case in the Phase II trials, they can do so again.

It is your duty to learn the truth and speak out—to stop the tragedy that is now taking place."

Excerpt from a letter by Dr Joan McKenna, Director of Research, TBM Associates, Berkeley California, which was published in the *Policy Review*, Fall, 1990: (see pages 90, 91)

"Like Duesberg and Ellison, we see the use of AZT as a political and economic solution without real medical benefit to the patients. AZT is a known immune suppressant that essentially shuts down the immune system. By administering AZT to AIDS and ARC patients, few symptoms emerge that require medical care or hospitalization until the final stage of massive system failure form multiple infections. With AZT, the insurance companies avoid the $150,000-$250,000 expenses of earlier AIDS cases where 9 to 18 months of hospital and medical care were threatening to bankrupt the companies. Hospital and health care administrators, including Medicaid officials, who saw their ruin looming as Medicaid AIDS patients filled their wards, were relieved that their financial exposure could be limited to a few weeks or months by AZT administration to patients. Politicians who were reluctant to expend more money and public resources for the care of economically and politically disenfranchised minorities could assuage concerned families and friends and the media that everything was being done that could be done medically with AZT. They promised to make AZT easier to obtain and require that all physicians seeing AIDS patients urge them to go on the drug. AZT does not stop the progression of the disease. It does not stop patients from dying. But the dying is quiet, convenient, and cheap at $5,000 to $15,000 per patient."

A report in the *New Scientist*, 19 October 1991 read: "Britain and France are to continue for at least another nine months a trial of the anti-AIDS drug Zidovudine (AZT) in which some participants receive only a placebo. The trial is designed to show whether the drug prolongs the lives of people infected with HIV but not showing symptoms of AIDS. But the US stopped a similar trial two years ago because the drug had already been shown to delay the progression of AIDS."

In February 1992 the trial, conducted by the Wellcome Pharmaceutical Company and the National Center for HIV Epidemiology and Clinical Research, was terminated for the same reasons given for the termination of the American trial, ie that it showed early AZT to benefit HIV-positive people, and so it would have been immoral to further withhold the drug from the placebo subjects.

Again, this is an example of "science by press release" (*The Australian*, 4 February 1992) because "it would be some time before the trial was published and a full assessment made", while in the meanwhile, the author was informed by the Sydney AIDS Centre, the data was held by the Wellcome Company as classified information. What will the full assessment reveal, seeing that the entire trial was based on pure supposition from start to finish? When it is known that less than 3% of HIV-positive people proceed to AIDS anyway, it is ridiculous to base a "scientific" trial on the basis that 100% will do so.

Of course, if Wellcome succeed in convincing everyone that AZT can save people from something that wouldn't have happened anyway, look at the sales they will make. The chairman of the trials advisory committee said the Wellcome Company had a moral obligation to drop its price for the drug (currently $5000–$9000 per patient per annum) now that it is proposed to give it to *all* HIV-positive people (15,000 in Australia alone), but the company has stated there will be no price reduction.

AZT is still the recommended treatment for AIDS, however, and now two new drugs are on the scene— Didanosine by Bristol-Myers, and Nevirapine by

Boehringer-Ingelheim, both of which are designed to destroy the "deadly" AIDS virus, HIV, against which in the eight years since it was accused, no evidence has been produced to show it does the slightest harm.

That the US Food and Drug Administration (FDA) has for years been a powerful instrument manipulated by the pharmaceutical companies has been obvious to some people for a long time. Its legislation has always been to stamp out as quackery all forms of natural therapies while at the same time protecting the interests of the drug manufacturers. In the US the FDA faces a bitter opponent in the form of the National Health Federation, dedicated to freedom of choice and the breaking of the medical monopoly which has become more and more profit motivated and, at the same time, counterproductive to public health. The NHF's journal *Health Freedom News*, October 1991 issue featured an opening article by the Federation's president, Maureen Salaman, titled "Watchdogs to Watch the FDA Watchdogs, Can the Food and Drug Administration Stand Close Scrutiny?" It commenced:

"Supposedly a reformer, FDA Commissioner David A Kessler, MD, continues ever-enduring FDA policy of giving undivided attention to a pimple and ignoring a cancer, of overlooking major pharmaceutical companies' toxic, sometimes lethal, drugs and persecuting small manufacturers of harmless vitamin supplements. Pursuing the same FDA course of letting the Goliaths of the drug industry get away with—yes—murder . . .

. . . Now what are Dr Kessler's ignored cancers? The antiquated, riddled-with-faults, rotten-with-politics approval system for harmful medicines and drugs, the FDA's hierarchy manned in many instances by former drug company executives—the revolving door system of executives flowing from the FDA into drug companies and vice-versa—and the FDA's Big Brother policy of arbitrarily raiding plants of legitimate nutritional supplement companies—intentionally or unintentionally keeping health-giving products off the market.

First things first. Anyone who has even glanced casually at an ad for a drug product in a medical magazine and noted the frightening side effects will feel icicles racing up and down their spine.

At best, any medicine or drug listed in the Physicians Desk Reference (PDR) *can sicken, disable, or even kill a patient while alleviating his symptoms. So prescribing any of them is potentially like playing catch with vials of nitroglycerine."*

And that's only the start of the article—and you can't say things like that in the USA unless you can back them up. And she does.

In conclusion to this chapter I should again emphasize that there are many medical drugs capable of destructive effects like those of AZT. Alpha interferon, the new drug recommended for the treatment of hepatitis C, has as previously mentioned the following side effects: depression, skin rashes and low white blood cell count. Great drug— it can pull you out of the minor league and make you eligible for AZT!

Thank God for the Salvation Army and the National Health Federation! (N.H.F. address: 212 W. Foothill Blvd, Monrovia, California 91017, P.O. Box 688 Monrovia)

Postscript on AZT

Science by Press Release
Within the space of one month several news reports about the AZT trials appeared in Australian newspapers, headlined as follows:

"EARLY AZT DOSES HALVE AIDS CASES"
              (The *Australian*, 4 February 1992)
"AZT NO SURVIVAL BENEFIT TO AIDS"
              (The *Courier Mail*, 14 February 1992)

"AIDS WONDER DRUG[4] FAILS TO PROLONG LIFE OF SUFFERERS"

(The *Australian*, 2 March 1992)

What Burroughs Wellcome and the FDA want everybody to believe from the first report is that even though AZT is destructive to the immune system, it is at the same time capable of slowing such destruction by its effect of arresting HIV activity if it is used early enough. In regard to the other reports, the AIDS establishment says that AZT treatment should have been started earlier, but nevertheless while lives were not prolonged, the patients were spared the worst symptoms before their final decline. So goes the old saying: "The operation was a success, but unfortunately the patient died." Cancer never gets a mention.

The realistic viewpoint of these reports is completely different. The Duesberg/Roote–Bernstein viewpoint is that the toxic effects of AZT given to symptom-free HIV-positive subjects actually assists the development of AIDS in many of them, and that the 50% who reportedly escaped did so because their constitutions were strong enough to combat the AZT toxicity. In other words they escaped, not because of AZT, but in spite of it. In relation to the reports about no survival benefit, the same argument applies, which is that many of the patients that perished would not have done so at all had they not been brainwashed (along with their doctors) to expect death, and then assisted to die by AZT poisoning.

Such discrepancies in the interpretation of observed phenomena need not imply conscious criminal intent by one party or another. More likely it demonstrates Dr William Roe's observations quoted in Chapter 6 which end:

"Indeed it seems the most destructive (and perhaps the most dangerous) characteristic of that species

---

[4] The license to call drugs "wonder drugs" is apparently a journalistic one, the product of a wild imagination.

of the genus *Homo* we conceitedly label *Sapiens* is not his wisdom but his reluctance to admit ignorance.

Rather than do so, he is prone to prosit an hypothesis and, all too frequently in the absence of supporting evidence, comes to believe it. Thus are myths created.''

Which is myth and which is fact in the argument on AIDS? If the reader is in doubt, perhaps the following chapter may assist in resolving it.

CHAPTER 10

Modern Medicine: A Snare and a Delusion

Futile but otherwise harmless medical care is the least important of the damages a proliferating medical enterprise inflicts on contemporary society. However, the pain, dysfunction, disability, and anguish resulting from techical medical intervention now rival the morbidity due to traffic and industrial accidents and even war-related activities, and make the impact of medicine one of the most rapidly spreading epidemics of our time.

Ivan Illich, *Medical Nemesis* (1976)

I believe my generation of doctors will be remembered for two things: the miracles that turned to mayhem, such as penicillin and cortisone, and for the millions of mutilations which are ceremoniously (and totally unnecessarily) carried out every year in operating rooms.

Robert A. Mendelsohn, MD
Confessions of a Medical Heretic (1979)

"Health care" is a modern term used by community leaders and doctors to describe a system which is the very opposite of health care, and which demonstrates mankind's greatest illusion: the belief you can make a sick person well by giving them medicine of some kind. The "quality" of health care is measured by our civic leaders in dollars—dollars— to pay for drugs, to develop new and better drugs, to pay the doctors who administer the drugs and to pay for hospitals in which the "care" can be administered. Money can buy care all right, but it is not health care.

An example of medical thinking is the recent report from the Australian Government Economic Planning Advisory Committee, which revealed that poor people on the average die ten years earlier than high income earners, are four times more likely to get respiratory diseases and other illnesses, and that they were twice as likely to die of cancer. The inference of this report was that poor people would not suffer so much if they had enough money to afford better health care. Of course you could just as easily conclude that germs get more fun out of seeking out and attacking poor people, but is it not more likely that a lot of poor people get sick, not because they are poor but because the same lack of capacity that keeps them poor keeps them also in total dietary ignorance?

A great deal of ingenuity goes into modern medicine, but not a great deal of intelligence. It takes a lot of ingenuity to devise the intricate procedures for a coronary bypass or transplant or reaming out blocked arteries, but why not tell the patient of the possibility of clearing blocked arteries by natural means—by strict diet? Why allow a recovering heart patient to eat a high-fat, high-cholesterol meal while still in coronary care?

Why are researchers looking for the "defective gene" which they say causes diabetes when it has been known at least as far back as 1936 that the prime cause of diabetes is a diet high in fat and protein, and that most diabetics produce all the insulin they need except that the insulin cannot work properly in a toxic bloodstream? And that on a proper diet most diabetics can be free of medical treatment in just a few weeks?

Why do some doctors state that arthritis and multiple

sclerosis are auto-immune diseases that happen when white cells go mad and attack their own domicile, while others blame retro-viruses and work to devise ways of thwarting their destructive "attacks"? These opinions are only supposition. Why don't doctors know that if you clear a patient's bloodstream of toxemia their white cells return to normal, that arthritis goes away, that MS goes "into remission", that blood pressure diminishes, ulcers heal, gallstones dissolve, migraines cease and so on?

The reason doctors do not know these simple facts is that standard medical training is based still on the medieval belief that diseases are "things" with evil intent that attack innocent people and that these things have to be counterattacked and driven out. Such beliefs are unacceptable to an intelligent observer and it is no wonder the "practice" of medicine is such a confused and fragmented affair.

It has been reported that from the ranks of doctors come the highest rates of suicides and drug dependency of all the occupations in society. Does this mean that doctors are more likely than others to become disillusioned and unhappy, that the career which once promised so much satisfaction at the start turns sour when the promise is not fulfilled? How many doctors, after working so hard to gain their qualifications, come to realize they have become little more than licensed drug pushers for the international drug cartels?

Many such doctors have reacted positively to set things right but usually they are considered eccentrics who are out to spoil a good set-up, and their complaints are ignored. Rejected and derided by their peers, a lot of them write books to get their message out of the barricade surrounding the medical profession, direct to the public. As books like these are written with great dedication and are based on direct observations made through the course of long medical careers, they make the best reading a medical student could get, but of course none are to be found in medical libraries anywhere.

A hundred years ago Dr Emmet Densmore and his

wife, also a medical doctor, collaborated to write a book called *How Nature Cures*. In this book the fallacies surrounding orthodox medicine were exposed, and to support his opinions Dr Densmore quoted some of the prominent physicians of the time who, like the Densmores, had awakened to the fact that orthodox medicine for the treatment of common diseases was a waste of effort bordering on the farcical. A few of the quotations were:
Professor Alonzo Clark, New York College of Physicians and Surgeons:

> "In their zeal to do good, physicians have done much harm. They have hurried thousands to the grave who would have recovered if left to Nature."

John Mason Good, MD FRS:

> "The efforts of medicine on the human system are in the highest degree uncertain, except indeed, that they have destroyed more lives than war, pestilence and famine combined."

Dr Eliphalet Kimball:

> "There is doctorcraft as well as priestcraft . . . Physicians have slain more than war. An instrument of death in their hands, bleeding, calomel, and other medicines have done more than powder and ball. The public would be infinitely better off without professed physicians. In weak constitutions Nature can be assisted. Good nursing is necessary, and sometimes roots and herbs do good. In strong constitutions medicine is seldom needed in sickness. To a man with a good constitution, and guided by reason in his course of living, sickness would be impossible."

Professor Alexander H. Stevens, New York College of Physicians and Surgeons:

> "The older physicians grow, the more skeptical they become of the virtues of medicine, and the more they are disposed to trust to the powers of Nature."

Sir John Forbes:

> "Some patients get well with the aid of medicines, some without, and still more in spite of it."

There were a great many other such quotations, the most descriptive of the situation being the one from the great physician and physiologist Professor Francois Magendie, President of the French Academy of Science:

> "Let us no longer wonder at the lamentable want of success which marks our practise, when there is scarcely a sound physiological principle among us. I hesitate not to declare, no matter how sorely I should wound our vanity, that so gross is our ignorance of the real nature of the physiological disorder called disease, that it would perhaps be better to do nothing, and resign the complaint into the hands of Nature, than to act as we are frequently compelled to do, without knowing the why and wherefore of our conduct, at the obvious risk of hastening the end of the patient.
>
> Gentlemen, medicine is a great humbug. I know it is called a science. Science indeed! It is nothing like science. Doctors are merely empirics when they are not charlatans. We are as ignorant as men can be. Who knows anything in the world about medicine? Gentlemen, you have done me a great honor to come here to attend my lectures, and I must tell you frankly now, in the beginning, that I know nothing in the world about medicine, and I don't know anybody who does know anything about it . . . I repeat, nobody knows anything about medicine . . .
>
> We are collecting facts in the right spirit, and I dare say, in a century or so, the accumulation of facts may enable our successors to form a medical science. Who can tell me how to cure the headache, or the gout, or disease of the heart? Nobody. Oh, you tell me the doctors cure people. I grant you people are cured, but how are they cured?

Gentlemen, Nature does a great deal, imagination
a great deal; doctors—devilishly little when they
don't do any harm.''

Frank statements, made a hundred years ago. Since
then, it is claimed, medicine has indeed become a science—
or has it? If Doctor Magendie were alive today and were
to inquire "Who can tell me how to cure the headache,
or the gout, or the disease of the heart?" he would be forced
again to conclude—nobody. Doctors can drug the
symptoms of headache, gout, heart disease and most other
complaints, but the patients are not cured, and many of
them die prematurely as a result of the drugs.

The fact of the matter is there is not, and cannot ever
be, such a thing as a medical "cure" for anything. Only
Nature can heal, but in their ignorance of this fact doctors
still continue to hopefully pour into their patients the drugs
recommended to them by the real controllers of the big
medical show, the drug companies.

In 1973, doctors in Israel went on strike and reduced
their total daily patient contacts from 65,000 to only 7000.
The strike lasted a month and during that time the death
rate, according to the Jerusalem Burial Society, dropped
fifty per cent. In 1976 in Bogota, Columbia, doctors refused
to treat all except emergency cases for a period of fifty-
two days, and in that time the death rate fell by thirty-
five per cent. In the same year, during a "slow-down" by
doctors in Los Angeles, the death rate there dropped
eighteen per cent. Obviously, Dr Densmore's opinions are
still valid today.

Headaches, gout, heart disease, cancer, hypertension,
diabetes, arthritis, MS, osteoporosis, premenstrual tension,
asthma, the common cold, herpes, AIDS—the list goes on—
all incurable still regardless of the claims and promises
of "medical science". Transplanting hearts, kidneys and
livers cannot be called curing; pumping insulin into
diabetics who are diabetic only because of their high-
protein, high-fat diet is not a cure either, nor is cutting
out a tumor and hoping like hell another will not take

its place. Despite 20th-Century technology and the admirable advances in lifesaving surgery and "crisis" medicine, for the most part modern medicine has advanced hardly at all in the last one hundred years in regard to solving the problem of common diseases. In fact there are more common diseases today than there ever were, and the list is growing.

Medicine is in a rut pointing the wrong way. The medical profession, like any other profession, contains only a few outstanding individuals out of a great multitude, all doing the best they can according to the way they have been trained. For some doctors medicine is a labor of love, while to others it is merely a lucrative and prestigious career. One way or another, in the status quo of society doctors have secured a highly favored niche, and like others so favored are not likely to welcome any form of change. Thus medicine is an extremely conservative profession, and not being answerable to higher authority it can cover up its shortcomings and run as a protected monopoly, virtually a law unto itself.

Doctors, over the past hundred years and despite their constant failures, have contrived to create the impression their services are of indispensable value; they have become so highly organized and influential that they have further contrived government legislation which protects them from competition under the pretext that they are protecting the public from charlatans. These achievements have been gained by the various medical associations which are the most powerful unions in the world and which, knowingly or unknowingly, have allowed the practice of medicine to become the drug-oriented pawn of the drug companies.

Mesmerised by the continuous flow of propaganda from the multibillion dollar drug companies, the ordinary hard-working doctor, knowing almost nothing about the etiology of disease, has become an innocent drug pusher in danger of getting writer's cramp from scribbling out prescriptions.

To what extent the average doctor realizes how farcical the situation really is in relation to treating disease would be difficult to ascertain, but one way or another the public deception is maintained. Medicine men, both primitive and modern, maintain with varying degrees of success an air of competence and mystique which sets them apart from ordinary people and disguises the fact they are quite ordinary people too, with human shortcomings and inner doubts. How is this gigantic deception maintained? It is maintained mainly by virtue of the fact that the healing power of Nature is so powerful. People actually recover in most cases in spite of the medical treatment they receive, and the chronically sick struggle to stay alive despite the drugs pumped into them. The illusion is that whatever good has eventuated has been achieved by the medicine, and of course when someone in pain is relieved of the pain by medicine at least some credit must be paid to drugs even if their side effects are damaging. But as Dr Ronald Glasser says in his book *The Body is the Hero*, the real healing is achieved by the body itself, while the doctor gets the credit.

Books like Dr Glasser's put the true perspective on modern medicine. There are many others on the topic that would put the fear of death in you, perhaps the most informative one on the subject being *Confessions of a Medical Heretic* by Doctor Robert S. Mendelsohn of Chicago (Contemporary Books, Chicago, 1979).

Dr Mendelsohn was in medical practice for over thirty-five years; he was Chairman of the Medical Licensing Committee of the State of Illinois and the recipient of numerous awards for excellence in medicine and medical instruction. At the time of writing his book he was the Associate Professor of Preventive Medicine at the University of Illinois, and in the introduction to his book he had this to say:

> "I do not believe in Modern Medicine, I am a medical heretic. My aim in this book is to persuade you to become a heretic, too.
>
> I haven't always been a medical heretic. I once believed in Modern Medicine.

In medical school, I failed to look deeply into a study that was going on around me, of the effects of the hormone DES—because I believed. Who could have suspected that twenty years later we would discover that DES causes vaginal cancer and genital abnormalities in children born to women receiving the drug during pregnancy?

I confess that I failed to be suspicious of oxygen therapy for premature infants, even though the best equipped and most advanced premature nurseries had an incidence of partial or total blindness of around ninety per cent of all low birth weight infants. A few miles away, in a large, less "advanced" hospital, the incidence of this condition—retrolental fibroplasia—was less than ten per cent. I asked my professors in medical school to explain the difference. And I believed them when they said the doctors in the poorer hospital just didn't know how to make the correct diagnosis.

A year or two later it was proved that the cause of retrolental fibroplasia was the high concentrations of oxygen administered to the premies. The affluent medical centers had higher rates of blinding simply because they could afford the very best nursery equipment: the most expensive and modern plastic incubators which guaranteed that all the oxygen pumped in reached the infant. At the poorer nurseries, however, old-fashioned incubators were used. They looked like bathtubs with very loose metal lids. They were so leaky that it made very little difference how much oxygen was pumped in: not enough reached the infant to blind it.

I still believed when I took part in a scientific paper on the use of the antibiotic Terramycin in treating respiratory conditions in premature babies. We claimed there were no side-effects. Of course there weren't. We didn't wait long enough to find out that not only didn't Terramycin—or any other antibiotic—do much good for these infections, but that it—and other tetracycline antibiotics—left thousands of children with yellow-green teeth and tetracycline deposits in their bones.

And I confess that I believed in the irradiation of tonsils, lymph nodes, and the thymus gland. I believed my professors when they said that of course radiation was dangerous, but that the doses we were using were absolutely harmless.

Years later—around the time we found out that the "absolutely harmless" radiation sown a decade or two before was now reaping a harvest of thyroid tumors—I couldn't help wondering when some of my former patients came back with nodules of their thyroids: Why are you coming back to me? To *me*, who did this to you in the first place?

But I no longer believe in Modern Medicine.

I believe that despite all the super technology and elite bedside manner that's supposed to make you feel about as well cared for as an astronaut on the way to the moon, the greatest danger to your health is the doctor who practices Modern Medicine.

I believe that Modern Medicine's treatments for disease are seldom effective, and that they're often more dangerous than the diseases they're designed to treat.

I believe the dangers are compounded by the widespread use of dangerous procedures for non-diseases.

I believe that more than ninety per cent of Modern Medicine could disappear from the face of the earth—doctors, hospitals, drugs and equipment—and the effect on our health would be immediate and beneficial.

I believe that Modern Medicine has gone too far, by using in everyday situations extreme treatments designed for critical conditions.

Every minute of every day Modern Medicine goes too far, because Modern Medicine *prides itself* on going too far. A recent article, "Cleveland's Marvellous Medical Factory", boasted of the Cleveland Clinic's "accomplishments" last year: 2,980 open-heart operations, 1.3 million laboratory tests, 73,320 electrocardiograms, 7,770 full-body x-ray scans, 210,378 other radiologic studies, 24,368 surgical procedures.

Not one of these procedures has been proved to have the least little bit to do with maintaining or restoring health. And the article, which was published in the Cleveland Clinic's own magazine, fails to boast or even mention that any people were helped by any of this expensive extravagance. That's because the product of this factory is not health at all.

So when you go to the doctor, you're seen not as a person who needs help with his or her health, but as a potential market for the medical factory's products.

If you're pregnant, you go to the doctor and he treats you as if you're sick. Childbirth is a nine-month disease which must be treated, so you're sold on intravenous fluid bags, fetal monitors, a host of drugs, the totally unnecessary episiotomy, and— the top of the line product—the Caesarean delivery!

If you make the mistake of going to the doctor with a cold or the flu, he's liable to give you antibiotics, which are not only powerless against colds and flu but which leave you more likely to come down with worse problems.

If your child is a little too peppy for his teacher to handle, your doctor may go too far and turn him into a drug dependent.

If your new baby goes off his or her feed for a day and doesn't gain weight as fast as the doctor's manual says, he might barrage your breastfeeding with drugs to halt the natural process and make room in the baby's tummy for man-made formula, which is dangerous.

If you're foolish enough to make that yearly visit for a routine examination, the receptionist's petulance, the other patients' cigarette smoke, or the doctor's very presence could raise your blood pressure enough so that you won't go home empty-handed. Another life "saved" by antihypertensive drugs. Another sex life down the drain since more impotence is caused by drug therapy than by psychological problems.

If you're unfortunate enough to be near a hospital when your last days on earth approach, your doctor will make sure your $500-a-day deathbed has all the latest electronic gear with a staff of strangers to hear your last words. But since those strangers are paid to keep your family away from you, you won't have anything to say. Your last sounds will be the electronic whistle on the cardiogram. Your relatives *will* participate: they'll pay the bill.

No wonder children are afraid of doctors. They *know!* Their instincts for real danger are uncorrupted. Fear seldom actually disappears. Adults are afraid, too. But they can't admit it, even to themselves. What happens is we become afraid of something else. We learn to fear not the doctor but what brings us to the doctor in the first place: our body and its natural processes.

When you fear something, you avoid it. You ignore it. You shy away from it. You pretend it doesn't exist. You let someone else worry about it. This is how the doctor takes over. We let him. We say: I don't want to have anything to do with *this, my body and its problems,* doc. You take care of it, doc. Do what you have to do.

So the doctor does.

When doctors are criticized for not telling their patients about the side effects of the drugs they prescribe, they defend themselves on the grounds that the doctor-patient relationship would suffer from such honesty. That defense implies that the doctor-patient relationship is based on something other than knowledge. *It's based on faith.*

We don't say we *know* our doctors are good, we say we have *faith* in them. We *trust* them.

Don't think doctors aren't aware of the difference. And don't believe for a minute that they don't play it for all it's worth. Because what's at stake is the whole ball game, the whole ninety per cent of more of Modern Medicine that we don't need, that, as a matter of fact, is out to kill us.

Modern Medicine can't survive without our faith, because Modern Medicine is neither an art nor a science. It's a religion.

One definition of religion identifies it as any organized effort to deal with puzzling or mysterious things we see going on in and around us. The Church of Modern Medicine deals with the most puzzling phenomena: birth, death, and all the tricks our bodies play on us—and we on them—in between. In *The Golden Bough*, religion is defined as the attempt to gain the favor of 'powers superior to man, which are believed to direct and control the course of nature and of human life.'

If people don't spend billions of dollars on the Church of Modern Medicine in order to gain favor with the powers that direct and control human life, what do they spend it on?

Common to all religions is the claim that reality is not limited to or dependent upon what can be seen, heard, felt, tasted or smelled. You can easily test modern medical religion on this characteristic by simply asking your doctor *why?* enough times. Why are you prescribing this drug? Why is this operation going to do me any good? Why do I have to do that? Why do you have to do that to me? Just ask *why?* enough times and sooner or later you'll reach the Chasm of Faith. Your doctor will retreat into the fact that you have no way of knowing or understanding all the wonders he has at his command. *Just trust me.*

You've just had your first lesson in medical heresy. Lesson Number Two is that if a doctor ever wants to do something to you that you're afraid of and you ask *why?* enough times until he says Just Trust Me, what you're to do is turn around and put as much distance between you and him as you can, as fast as your condition will allow.

Unfortunately, very few people do that. They submit. They allow their fear of the witch doctor's mask, the unknown spirit behind it, and the mystery of what is happening and of what will happen, to change into respectful awe of the whole show.

But you don't have to let the witch doctor have his way. You can liberate yourself from Modern Medicine—and it doesn't mean you'll have to take chances with your health. In fact, you'll be taking less of a chance with your health, because there's no more dangerous activity than walking into a doctor's office, clinic, or hospital *unprepared.* And by *prepared* I don't mean having your insurance forms filled out. I mean you have to get in and out alive *and* accomplish your mission. For that, you need appropriate tools, skills, and cunning.

The first tool you must have is knowledge of the enemy. Once you understand Modern Medicine as a religion, you can fight it and defend yourself much more effectively than when you think you're fighting an art or a science. Of course, the Church of Modern Medicine never calls itself a church. You'll never see a medical building dedicated to the religion of medicine, always to medical *arts* or medical *science.*

Modern Medicine relies on faith to survive. All religions do. So heavily does the Church of Modern Medicine rely on faith that if everyone somehow simply forgot to believe in it for just one day, the whole system would collapse. For how else could any institution get people to do the things Modern Medicine gets people to do, without inducing a profound suspension of doubt? Would people allow themselves to be artificially put to sleep and then cut to pieces in a process they couldn't have the slightest notion about—if they didn't have faith? Would people swallow the thousands of tons of pills every year—again without the slightest knowledge of what these chemicals are going to do—if they didn't have faith?

If Modern Medicine had to validate its procedures objectively, this book wouldn't be necessary. That's why I'm going to demonstrate how Modern Medicine is not a church you want to have faith in.

Some doctors are worried about scaring their patients. While you're reading this book, you are, in a sense, my patient. I think you *should* be scared. You're supposed to be scared when your well-being and freedom are threatened. And you are, right now, being threatened.

If you're ready to learn some of the shocking things your doctor knows but won't tell you; if you're ready to find out if your doctor is dangerous; if you're ready to learn how to protect yourself from your doctor; you should keep reading, because that's what this book is about.

And that's just the beginning of Dr Mendelsohn's book.

There are many other similar books written by dedicated doctors like Dr Mendelsohn; a more recent one by Dr Stuart M. Berger called *What Your Doctor Didn't Learn in Medical School* (Bantam, 1988) describes frightening reports of doctor-induced illness among hospital patients (thirty-six per cent of patients in one hospital), among which illnesses was serious kidney damage caused by antibiotics. He said it was estimated that as many as four million hospital-induced infections may occur each year in the US, meaning that "108,000 Americans will die—either entirely or in part due to the infections they acquired courtesy of the medical machine". Dr Berger said:

> "I recall one day in medical school, shortly after I began making rounds on the wards, having a sinking revelation: that hospitals, just like any other human enterprise, are just a vast interlocking constellation of human foibles, frailties and failings. People make mistakes, confusion abounds, politics fester, neglect occurs, greed persists. Things are, in short, no different than in a corporation, a neighborhood, or a Boy Scout troop. The stakes are just higher."

That the practice of medicine is in fact on the whole counterproductive to its professed purpose is a situation that makes the Watergate Scandal look like a kids' party, but who can demolish an institution that is more ingrained in human culture than organized crime and high level corruption? People believe in medicine, they want medicine—it promises so much for so little (your life in exchange for your life's savings)—so while they continue being hooked on savory food and other indulgences, the majority will continue to accept the diseases ingrained in our culture and take their medicine until they are cured to death.

The Future of Medicine

There are signs that a gradual awareness of the importance of nutrition is dawning within the medical profession, an awareness forced upon it by persevering people like Nathan Pritikin. In 1982 a comprehensive report called *Diet, Nutrition and Cancer* was issued by the US National Research Council. The report was prepared by a committee of people from the National Academy of Science, the

National Academy of Engineering and the Institute of Medicine. Although the report revealed a lamentable lack of comprehension of the subject, it did in fact demonstrate that nutrition was a significant factor in the origins of cancer. Note that the report emanated from outside the medical profession, as has a recently released book in Australia called *Diet, Health and Disease in Australia*, written by a number of doctors and produced by the Australian Academy of Science.

The research for both of these books obviously did not extend far outside conventional circles. In relation to cancer the lack of knowledge was lamentable, as was the lack of knowledge of diabetes and other disease problems described in the Australian book.

Inadequate as these books may be, it is gratifying that they have appeared at all; it shows that some doctors are at last breaking free of their mental shackles.

In his book *Man The Unknown*, the great physician and philosopher Alexis Carrel said: "Unless the doctors of today become the dieticians of tomorrow then the dieticians of today will become the doctors of tomorrow." Maybe this is starting to happen. Evolution is a slow process, and bearing in mind that it took hundreds of years for people to accept that the world was round, I suppose we should not complain too much.

In Defense of Doctors

In criticising others one must always put oneself in their position and remember: "There but for the grace of God go I." And so in defense of doctors with all their ignorance of the "outside world", this chapter concludes with an explanation by Dr G. T. Wrench of England contained in the introduction to his book *The Wheel of Health*, published in 1938:

> It should be clearly understood that a doctor is one
> so saturated with people's illnesses and ailments

that, if thoughtful, he is almost forced to look upon life as something heavily burdened by these defects.

I shall myself carry with me the profound impression of the first months I spent in the hospital wards and out-patient departments many years ago. I had come from the vigorous and exuberant life of an English public school, where everything that really absorbed one's boyish interests was based on a glowing vitality and responsive health. After the penance of school hours there was plenty of time to let the muscles go—games, sports, ragging, bathing, or running and walking over untilled fields. All these things were in sunlight and wind or the raw cold, which made the blood snap round its course.

Something of this life accompanies the early years of the medical student, but there is always about one the lure of the hospital work to draw one to its consuming interests. One is caught in the meshes of the problems of disease, from which one will not be able to free the mind for the rest of one's life. For impressions of youth are those that remain. They color all one's thoughts and experience, they largely select that thought and experience. And the impression of the quantity of diseases and the suffering due to them is a tremendous one. I used sometimes to walk about London with my eyes down and with the question "Why?" upon my lips until I saw pictures of the many maleficent objects of pathology upon the pavements, so vivid was the impression which the microscope and the post-mortem room made upon me.

The effect was not one of depression; that is not the effect upon healthy youth. It was one which stimulated one like a stouter opponent than oneself at boxing. Here was truly a prodigious opponent, the problem of disease, why man is so affected.

After debating the question—Why disease? Why not health?—again and again with my fellow

students, I slowly, before I qualified, came to a
further question—Why was it that as students we
were always presented with sick or convalescent
people for our teaching and never with the ultra-
healthy? Why were we only taught disease? Why
was it presumed that we knew all about health in
its fullness? The teaching was wholly one-sided.
Moreover, the basis of our teaching upon disease
was pathology, namely, the appearance of that
which is dead from disease.

We started from our knowledge of the dead,
from which we interpreted the manifestations, slight
or severe, of threatened death, which is disease.
Through these various manifestations, which
fattened our text-books, we approached health. By
the time, however, we reached real health, like that
of the keen times of public school, the studies
were dropped. Their human representatives, the
patients, were now well, and neither we nor our
educators were any longer concerned with them.
We made no studies of the healthy—only the sick.

Disease was the reason for our specialized
existences. There was also a great abundance of it.
Between its abundance and its need to ourselves its
inevitability was taken for granted. Gradually,
however, a question forced itself upon me more and
more insistently. Had not some of this 'inevitability'
attached to disease come about by our profession
only viewing disease from within? What would
happen if we reversed the process and started by
learning all we could about the healthiest people
and animals whom we could discover? This
question pursued me with considerable constancy,
but unfortunately I was not provided with that will
which is a part of which I reverence so much—
the genius of discovery. Those who possess it grip
an idea and never let it go. They are as passionate
for it to get on in the world as the mother is for
her offspring; daring, as even weak animals do, to

challenge hopeless odds on its behalf. After
achieving a small local repute in research, all I did
was to apply for scholarships, and in my
applications I placed a subject of my own choice,
to study the health of the healthiest people I could
discover.

I did not, of course, succeed. My proposal was
probably looked upon as ridiculous. To research
in health was a complete reversal of the accustomed
outlook, which was confined by the nature of the
profession to different aspects of disease. For to the
profession disease is the base and substance of its
structure and health just the top of the pyramid,
where it itself comes to an end. To propose reversing
this was like asking one to stand on one's head
to get the right point of view.

At any rate my applications came to nothing,
though I was offered work upon the accepted lines.
In this I had not the necessary faith, so I gave up
research and went into practice. I remained
interested in very healthy people and read what I
could about them, but the work imposed by the
war and by practice in the following years withheld
me from anything more than an academic interest
in the old question—Health; why not?

It was not until two years ago, when I had
more leisure, that a vivid sentence in the writings
of Sir Robert McCarrison thawed my frozen hope.
The sentence was: 'These people are unsurpassed
by any Indian race in perfection of physique; they
are long lived, vigorous in youth and age, capable
of great endurance and enjoy a remarkable freedom
from disease in general.' Further study of his
writings was very encouraging. Here was a research
worker who researched in health and healthy
people; in fact he presented to himself health as
a problem, and produced answers to it, in some
such words as the following: 'Here is a people of
unsurpassed health and physique, and here are
researches into the reasons thereof.'

In this way it will be seen we come as researchers straight to health without intervention, and to health in the full dictionary sense of the word of wholeness, namely, sound physique of every organ of the body without exceptions and freedom from disease. This is the knowledge which we all want to know. We want to know what is full health, whether the tremendous part illness and ailments play in modern civilized countries is really necessary and, if not, upon what primarily does health depend. We can ourselves attain to health—or at least with our modern skill in investigation we should be able to do so—if this full health exists in any part of our Empire today. We shall at least learn more about how to be healthy ourselves and how to bring healthy children into the world by studying successful human examples than we can by any other way.

By studying the wings of birds in flight we have made our machines carry us through the air. By studying one of the healthiest peoples of the world we might so improve our methods of health as to become a really healthy people ourselves. A research in health is really promising. Well, here is one. Let us see if the promise is fulfilled."

Having presented Dr Wrench's point of view, it should be noted that this chapter, which so severely criticizes the modern practice of medicine, is composed entirely from the observations and opinions of doctors and scientists. It concludes the same way, with the statements of four of the most distinguished physicians of the 20th Century.

Dr William Roe (retired) of Nelson, New Zealand, the author of *Science in Medical Practise* (1984) in which he strongly criticises modern medicine, said this:

"By starting from a false premise, a superstructure has been created which is, to a not inconsiderable degree, an iatrogenic[1] fantasy. The primary function

---

[1] Iatric: relating to medicine or physicians. Iatrogenic: induced by medical treatment.

of medicine has been transformed from a service to patients to a vocation and avocation for medical and paramedical personnel; iatrogenic disease has become a major problem and medicine has become big business. An urgent need exists to correct this imbalance, to restore the art of medicine to its former status."

Dr Maynard Murray, B.Sc MD, Fort Myers Florida, from his book *Sea Energy Agriculture* (1976):

"Are we kidding ourselves with longevity statistics and 'war against disease' statistics? You bet we are!

Our medical statistics equate the increasing in the average lifespan with good health. This kind of reasoning makes appealing newscopy, but it reminds me of the statistician who drowned in a river with an average depth of one foot. Such propaganda is deathly deceiving. This specious reasoning can lull us into a feeling of unwarranted wellbeing.

I promise not to belabor this negative approach much longer, but it seems we Americans, collectively, are a lot like the Mexican burro that requires a smack between the eyes with a two by four plank before attention is focussed . . ."

Dr Kasper Blond, of England (referring specifically to cancer):

"The problem of cancer must be considered as an insoluble medical problem because it is essentially a nutritional and social problem;[2] in other words, a problem of prevention.

Such a problem cannot be solved by animal experiments, vaccines and drugs. Statisticians, pathologists, biochemists and doctors cannot solve social problems."

And finally to repeat the great Dr Alexis Carrel:

---

[2] As are all the rest.

"Unless the doctors of today become the dieticians
of tomorrow, then the dieticians of today will
become the doctors of tomorrow."

The time that elapses between the introduction of an
innovative idea and its general acceptance in society is called
"the culture gap", and varies enormously with the amount
of publicity the new idea receives. If a lot of money hinges
on the outcome, powerful financial forces, motivated by
either the promise of gain or the fear of loss, can either
promote the idea or forcefully suppress it. Thus the culture
gap in women's fashions may be only a few weeks, and
in medicine perhaps a hundred years. But the latter gap
nevertheless is closing as the following report indicates:

A MEATLESS AMERICA BY THE YEAR 2050?
(Report by *Longevity Magazine*, June 1991)
The Physicians' Committee for Responsible
Medicine, Washington, DC is waging an all-out war
to scratch meat and dairy products from the four
basic food groups, long billed as a healthy diet.

The report went on to say that "a wealth of studies"
have linked meatless, low-fat, low-cholesterol, high-fiber
diets with low rates of cancer, heart disease and other life-
shortening conditions, but that it may take several decades
before the American public embraces a meatless diet. Dr
Neal Barnard, President of the Physicians' Committee
concluded: "But only twenty years ago, eating steak was
an enviable sign of affluence. Now when people eat red
meat, it's with a guilty conscience because they know it's
bad for you."

Note: The diet recommended by the Physicians'
Committee contains large quantities of grains and legumes
and very little fruit, much the same as the Pritikin diet,
and is therefore not recommended because of the adverse
effects of too much emphasis on grains and legumes.

Nevertheless, the Physicians' Committee for
Responsible Medicine is to be commended for their
breakaway from old, worn-out ideas and their adoption
of a fresh new attitude. Alexis Carrel would be pleased.

Postscript on Modern Medicine

If what you have already read about the poisoning effects of medical drugs, vaccinations, etc has not made you question which are the most dangerous—pharmaceutical drugs or germs—perhaps the following true story will.

The story is recounted from a recent edition of *The Australian Weekend Magazine* and is entitled "Ben's Story". It is the story of a twenty-two-year-old Queensland University 1st Class honours student awarded a $20,000 scholarship for research work in biometrics. To gain experience before commencing his doctorate he, with two other young male companions, embarked on a backpacking tour of Nepal, Thailand and Malaysia, a trip which was to end in disaster.

Lean and good-looking, Ben must have been very fit, having not long before this tour trekked around Tasmania and other parts of Australia as well as powering a pedicab around Brisbane all year showing tourists about in order to supplement his limited means. As his sister said:

> "Thorough as always, he packed only two changes of clothes in order to make room for a comprehensive medical kit containing antiseptic, dressings, antibiotics, burn cream and insect repellent.
>
> Malaria was just one of his many health concerns, and along with being immunized against typhoid, cholera, hepatitis B, polio and tetanus through the University of Queensland Health Service, he obtained prescriptions for Malofrim and Chloroquine, the recommended anti-malarial drugs."

According to one of his companions: "Ben was the one always on the ball with the drugs", nagging his friends to take theirs. "He was meticulous."

After about four weeks in Nepal and about five days in Ko Chang, a Thai island, the boys split up and Ben went by bus to Singapore. Seven days after leaving Ko Chang, Ben started getting alternating fevers and chills, which he put down to a flu-like virus he could not shake, and he arrived a few days later in Singapore after an all-night bus journey. Staying with friends, he slept most of the day of his arrival, and on the following day, complaining of "dark urine" and sore kidneys, he visited a doctor who diagnosed a possible kidney infection.

Later the same day he was admitted to Singapore General Hospital and soon afterwards his friends were alarmed by a phone call from the hospital informing them Ben was comatose with failed kidneys and suspected septicemia, a liver tumor or malaria. The following day he suffered cardiac arrest and was revived, only to pass away the following morning.

The medical verdict, based on the blood tests earlier done, was malaria,[3] because the malarial microbe *Plasmodium falciparum* was found. Over the same period of time, the companion who had shared a hut with Ben in Ko Chang had also come down with malaria and had spent two weeks in hospital in Penang before recovering well enough to travel home. Although Ben's friend could not recall being bitten by a mosquito in Ko Chang, it was natural enough to assume that they both had been, and suffered malaria as a result. That, you might agree, is a reasonable assumption.

Once upon a time the writer certainly would have agreed, but that was before I learned enough to write this book. That was before I watched my son die, having

---

[3] Medical authorities state that among Australian military personnel serving in New Guinea, the expected incidence of malaria is one person in five. Worldwide, the fatality rate was estimated to be 1.5 per cent of people contracting the disease.

The symptoms of severe anemia and dark-colored urine, sometimes called blackwater fever, and associated usually with the falciparum microbe, seldom occurred in people who had been in the malarial region for less than six months and who had not already suffered at least four previous attacks.

If this is the case, once again arises the question: does the pathological factor reside in the microbe or in the host?

displayed in hospital dark urine, fever and comatose after weeks of heavy "scientific" drug therapy.

When you consider a single course of penicillin and terramycin, designed to protect orphan children against infections, was sufficient to cause them pneumocystis carinii pneumonia (Chapter 7), and when you consider how supposedly harmless vaccinations for supposed protection against diptheria, whooping cough, tetanus, etc, can cause, within six weeks, symptoms of tuberculosis, chills, fever, meningitis and gastroenteritis with the concurrent presence of tubercule bacilli,[4] one is powerfully inclined to agree with Professor Oliver Wendell Holmes when he said: "If all the drugs were cast into the sea, it would be so much better for man, and so much the worse for the fishes."

When Ben felt his first symptoms of fever, etc commence, did he use his carefully prepared kit of antibiotics to try and allay them? That was the very purpose he carried the kit with him, so it is reasonable to assume he did.

The author, from the age of twenty-one through to fifty-three, travelled continually through New Guinea, the Pacific Isles, the Far East, Thailand, India, Pakistan, Egypt and the Middle East, in the days before hygiene and Hilton Hotels, never took any medicine and was bitten by many mosquitoes. I had a sore throat in Rome in 1958 and a touch of food poisoning in Singapore once in 1962. I didn't believe in medicine then, and I sure as hell don't now.

It is three years now since I lost my youngest son and I still feel the pain of grief, although of course it lessens with time. So I know how it feels and can sympathize with Ben's family.

May the loss of Mike and Ben help us to understand how better to protect ourselves, bearing in mind that in order to understand one must never blithely accept answers without first asking a lost of questions.

---

[4] *The Hazards of Immunization* (Sir Graham Wilson, MD, London, 1967).

CHAPTER 11

Heart Disease: Civilization's No. 1 Killer

With a cholesterol level of 150 [3.9 mmol/l] or less, plaque reversal in two years is possible.
Dr Robert Wissler, Chicago Medical School,
June 1977

The major cause of death in modern countries is atherosclerosis, the diseased state of the arteries which results in heart attacks, stroke, kidney failure and many other less lethal health problems. Because the most common direct cause of death is heart attack, great prominence has been given to heart disease, which term really only describes the local manifestation of atherosclerosis in the region of the heart and the coronary arteries which supply the heart muscle with blood. The heart muscle like any other muscle requires an adequate blood supply. When heart disease exists it is common for atherosclerosis to exist elsewhere in the body at the same time, in which case symptoms other than chest pains or heart attack may show up first. Such symptoms, all related, are high blood pressure (hypertension), stroke, kidney failure, claudication, glaucoma, premature senility and so on. All due to lipotoxemia derived from the Western diet.

Generally speaking, there are two forms of atherosclerosis, one in which the arteries become mineralized with calcium and lesser minerals, becoming hard and brittle (hardening of the arteries), and one in which the arteries absorb mushy deposits of fat and cholesterol and gradually become blocked with a porridge-like substance called atheroma. Hardening of the arteries used to be called arteriosclerosis and was more common many years ago when diets were based more on grain products and starchy vegetables. Nowadays atheroma is more common because the Western diet is based more on animal protein foods, dairy products, etc, containing large amounts of fat and cholesterol. Whether caused by one or both of these factors combined, the diseased state of arteries is today called atherosclerosis in medical circles.

As the disease progresses, and blood supply to various parts of the body begins to be curtailed, the body attempts to maintain the supply by growing many tiny blood vessels to form a bypass around the blocking sections of artery. These very fine vessels provide what is called "collateral circulation" which can be so effective that no symptoms of the potentially fatal situation are displayed—at least if the blood is thin enough (ie of low viscosity) to pass easily through the fine vessels. Should the blood become sticky, which can happen after one fatty meal or in a highly stressful situation, the collateral circulation will of course diminish or cease, the consequence of which will be increased "coronary deficiency" displayed by chest pain called angina or perhaps by injury to the heart muscle called "heart attack". When circulation to the lower limbs is similarly curtailed, muscle pains are experienced and walking affected, a condition called claudication. Diminished circulation to the brain may be indicated by vagueness and premature senility, culminating as a stroke. And so on . . . it is all the same disease—atherosclerosis via lipotoxemia.

When coronary arteries become severely blocked, all it needs to precipitate a heart attack is for sticky blood or a clot at a critical point to block off circulation to part of the heart muscle, and the severity of the attack will depend on just how much of the heart muscle is affected. In some cases the heart muscle may gradually be depleted by a series of small attacks that pass almost unnoticed, and in other cases when a major coronary artery suddenly blocks the resultant attack may be massive and fatal. The most quickly fatal heart attack is one in which the heart's nervous centre is affected and the co-ordinated pumping action of the heart muscle suddenly changes to an unco-ordinated flutter called fibrillation.

In many such situations which in the ordinary course of events would be fatal, the heart can be restarted with prompt medical attention—in the case of the blood clot by the injection of streptokinase, an enzyme which dissolves blood clots, and in the case of fibrillation by an electric shock from a special defibrillator or even by physically thumping the patient's chest. This is "crisis medicine" at its best and is one reason that death rates from heart attacks have diminished in recent years, the main reasons however being that educated people are more diet conscious, smoke less and exercise more.

It seems incredible that the simple facts about heart disease are not more widely known, even among doctors, because they have been available for many years. For at least all the 20th Century it has been known that excessive amounts of animal protein foods in the diet lead to what was earlier known as cardiac-vascular-renal disease, but it was Dr Lester Morrison of Los Angeles who finally correlated fat and cholesterol factors in the modern diet with the growing epidemic of heart disease. The role of cholesterol in artery disease had been argued about since 1911, at which time Russian researchers had demonstrated that rabbits fed cholesterol developed blocked arteries, but the picture was confused because it was also known that carnivorous animals constantly eating cholesterol did not do so. That carnivores of course have different digestive systems to rabbits and eat their food raw apparently was not taken into account. Anyway, in the 1930s Dr Morrison was researching the relationship between alcohol consumption and cirrhosis of the liver, and was feeding animals with fats and cholesterol to produce cirrhosis in them, which it did, but at the same time he was amazed to observe that their coronary arteries blocked with atheroma just like the arteries of humans with heart disease.

Having proven to his own satisfaction that the worsening epidemic of heart disease was due to the high levels of fat and cholesterol in the Western diet, and knowing that dietary correction enabled heart patients to regain normal health and vigor, and knowing furthermore that such discoveries take years to penetrate the medical profession, if at all, Dr Morrison wrote a book to inform the public direct, as many other doctors have been forced to do. The book was called *The Low-Fat Way to Health and Longer Life* (Prentice-Hall, 1958).

It may seem superfluous to describe all these events, but there is a purpose. First, to illustrate how the best medical advice is never obtainable through conventional channels, and second, to show how one event leads to another, in this case the health career of Nathan Pritikin. Pritikin had been following Dr Morrison's work with great interest since 1946 and it was from their first meeting in 1955 that Pritikin realized he was himself in serious danger from heart disease, from which point he went on to develop the diet that bears his name and to devote the remaining years of his life to spreading the gospel of health.

Since that time it has been demonstrated scientifically that not only can atherosclerosis be prevented by proper diet,[1] but it can also be reversed.

Why, then, after all these years is heart disease still our No. 1 killer? It seems that the simple facts of life are still unknown to most people and their doctors, on top of which our traditional diet supplemented by junk food is an addiction too difficult to shake. Government funded health organizations like the National Heart Foundation do their best to educate the masses, but their out-of-date information is still advocating too many protein, fat and

[1] *See* "Mineral Deficiencies", Chapter 14 (Dr Maynard Murray's experiments with rabbits).

cholesterol foods. Conventional dietary advice is still based on the four basic food groups concept devised in 1956 by the US Department of Agriculture[2] and supported of course by the meat, dairy and cereal industries, thus leading the most conscientious people nutritionally astray.

Be that as it may, the answer to the problem of avoiding heart disease is not to eat the foods that cause atherosclerosis. Remember that all foods of animal origin, including dairy products and eggs, contain fat and cholesterol and too much protein. Lay off them and preferably avoid them. Replace them with fresh fruit and vegetables and don't make Pritikin's mistake of overindulging in grain products. Foods from vegetable sources contain no cholesterol, they contain proper amounts of protein and fats, and provide better nutrition with less toxic by-products if consumed uncooked. It is easier said than done, but is preferable to coronary bypass surgery. And of course if it is done properly there will be no toxemia and therefore no cancer, arthritis, diabetes and all the rest.

[2] In Australia the basic foods are divided into five separate groups.

CHAPTER 12

Cancer: Civilization's No. 2 Killer

There is no disease in existence which is, most assuredly, easier of prevention than cancer; yet there is no malady which, when once it has established its presence, is so difficult to subdue.

Robert Bell, MD FRFPS
Late Vice-president of the International Society of
Cancer Research
Late Superintendent of Cancer Research, Battersea
Hospital
Member, Cosmopolitan Society of Cancer Research

Cancer is a state of cellular growth which occurs when some normal cells in the body become abnormal and multiply abnormally. It is characterized by the ability of the abnormal cells to subdivide and multiply outside of the constraints that automatically limit the subdivision and growth of normal cells. It is resultant of imperfect blood chemistry and does not occur in properly nourished and vigorously healthy humans. While cancer is unknown among various primitive populations throughout the world, it is common in modern countries, being responsible for one in every four deaths, and is still increasing.

When the epidemiological facts are considered, even briefly, it becomes apparent that the "diseases of civilization", of which cancer is only one, are directly caused by faulty living habits practised by the supposedly more civilized populations, and when the different dietary and other living habits are compared, it soon becomes further apparent what the main faults are. And to understand how these faults (mainly dietary) lead to the chronic toxemia which provokes once-healthy cells to change form, only a rudimentary knowledge of elementary biology is required, together with the acceptance that all life forms are capable of adaptation to a changed environment if necessary for survival.

What Causes Cancer?

For a start, it has been proven that germs and viruses do not cause cancer. Present cancer research is working on the supposition that cancer is caused by toxins of various kinds which one way or another find their way into the body and in some locations cause damage to the nucleus of a cell, turning it into a cancer cell. The presumption is that a gene within the DNA structure of the cell becomes altered so that the cell begins to multiply. Such a change to the cell's DNA is called a mutation. Also suspected of being able to cause cancer in this way are various forms of radiation, and any substance or influence that either causes cancer or tends to cause cancer is called a carcinogen. This hypothesis is a simple one, and if it were true it should be easy to prove, but although it is well known that certain substances can be carcinogenic, they are not always so, and the mechanism by which they are supposed to work has never been demonstrated. The hypothesis therefore remains only guesswork, and in the minds of most doctors cancer remains a mystery.

However, there is a theory on the causation of cancer which has been proven—one which accords to all known facts and biological laws and has been demonstrated in the laboratory. This theory, called the De-differentiation Theory of Cancer, developed from knowledge accumulated about how aerobic cells generate energy by the respiration of oxygen, and is best explained in the books of four of the 20th Century's greatest medical scientists: Dr Otto Warburg, Dr Max Gerson of Germany, Dr William F. Koch of the USA, and Dr Cornelius Moerman of Holland.

Dr Otto Warburg (1883–1970) was Director of the Max Planck Institute of Cell Physiology in Germany. The holder of many international honors, Dr Warburg was considered by Dr Dean Burk, head of the Cytochemistry Department of the US National Cancer Institute at the time, to be the world's greatest biochemist. In 1931 Warburg won the Nobel Prize in Medicine for his discovery of the oxygen transferring enzyme of cell respiration, and was voted a second Nobel Prize in 1944 for his discovery of the active groups of the hydrogen transferring enzymes. Conferred honorary degrees by the universities of Harvard, Oxford and Heidelberg, he was a member of the Royal Society of London, a Knight of the Order of Merit founded by Frederick the Great, and was awarded the Great Cross with Star and Shoulder Ribbon of the Bundesrepublik. Although Jewish, he was unmolested by the Nazis, and in the subsequent invasion of Germany by the Russians he was accorded protection and special consideration by the Russian High Command. Warburg's research spanned more than sixty years, and he was the author of over 500 published research papers and five books. His description of the experiments in which he transformed normal cells into cancer cells was contained in his lecture at the meeting of Nobel-Laureates on 30 June 1966 at Lindau, Germany. This lecture, titled "The Prime Cause and Prevention of Cancer", was reproduced in English by Dr Dean Burk and published by Konrad Triltsch, Wurzburg, Germany.

Dr Dean Burk (1904–1988) was a foundation member of the US National Cancer Institute and former head of its Cytochemistry Department. For his work in cancer research he received honors from France, Britain, Germany and Russia. Formerly Associate Professor of Biochemistry, Cornell University, he worked in cancer research at the Kaiser Wilhelm Institute in Germany and at the USSR Academy of Science, Moscow. Dr Burk was the recipient

new discs - neck

287 - Horne

of the Domagk Prize for cancer research, a Knight Commander of the Medical Order of Bethlehem, and a Knight of the Mark Twain Society. He was co-author of the books *Cancer, Approaches to Tumor Chemotherapy* and *Cell Chemistry* and author of over 250 published scientific papers. Dr Warburg said Burk's outstanding and decisive discoveries in cancer research were: 1) the metabolism of the regenerating liver (1941); 2) that the malignancy of cancer was proportional to the fermentation rate of the cells (1956); and 3) that in vivo growing hepatomas produced in vivo by carcinogens were similarly more malignant the higher the fermentation rate (1964).

Dr Max Gerson (1881-1959) was Jewish but didn't enjoy Warburg's standing. He was forced to flee Germany in 1933, spending the last twenty odd years of his life working in the USA. Best known for his successful dietary treatment of migraine, lupus, tuberculosis, diabetes and cancer, Gerson was the author of more than fifty published research papers and four books. Whereas Warburg was supported and honored for his full-time research, Gerson's great work was ignored by the medical establishment. He worked alone devoting his efforts mainly to the treatment of his patients, most of whom had been given up as hopeless cases by other doctors. Under Gerson's care, Dr Albert Schweitzer, double Nobel Laureate, completely eliminated his diabetes and Schweitzer's wife her tuberculosis using Gerson's dietary methods. After Gerson's death Dr Schweitzer said of him: "I see in him one of the most eminent geniuses in the history of medicine." Notwithstanding recognition by such medical greats as Dr Schweitzer and Dr Ferdinand Sauerbruch, Gerson's work received no recognition by the medical establishment, which considered him an unorthodox threat to the medical system.

William F. Koch, BA MA Ph.D MD, was Instructor in Histology and Embryology at the University of Michigan from 1910-14, Professor of Physiology at the Detroit College of Medicine from 1914-19, and Director of the Koch Cancer Clinic from 1919-49. Like Gerson, Koch was considered unorthodox and a threat to the established medical system, and despite adoption of his methods by independent doctors in the USA and Canada, he was continually persecuted by the American Medical Association, run at the time by a criminal who called himself Dr Maurice Fishbein but whose medical credentials were false. (Fishbein's dictatorial control of American medicine finally ended when he was kicked out at the AMA Convention in Atlantic City on 6 June 1949.) Koch was author of numerous publications concerned primarily with the biochemistry of immunity and of cancer, his best-known book being *The Survival Factor in Neoplastic and Viral Diseases*, published in 1961. Dr Willard Dow, founder of the Dow Chemical Company, described Dr Koch as the greatest biochemist of the age and so far ahead of his contemporaries that they could not understand him.

Dr Cornelius Moerman graduated in medicine in 1930 and since then has devoted his entire professional life to cancer research and treatment. His theory of cancer, which he called the Metabolism Theory, he developed independently, but because his reasoning was based on the new knowledge about the respiratory processes of cells and the enzymes necessary for their accomplishment, his conclusions of course inevitably coincided with those of Warburg, Gerson and Koch. The English translation of his book *A Solution to the Cancer Problem* was published in 1962 by The International Association of Cancer Victims and Friends Inc., Los Angeles.

Although doctors Gerson, Koch and Moerman each separately arrived at the same conclusion and demonstrated the theory by their successful treatment of human patients, it was Dr Warburg who demonstrated visually in the laboratory the actual changing of normal cells into cancer cells.

In fact, Dr Warburg was not the first to demonstrate that cancer arose from cells whose normal respiration had been disturbed. P.G. Seeger had proven this in 1936, 1937 and 1938 but it was F. Windisch in 1947 who succeeded in changing normal cells into cancer cells by intermittently withholding oxygen from them, an experiment repeated in 1953 by H. Goldblatt and G. Cameron. Dr Warburg's experiments, however, actually measured the degrees of respiration and fermentation involved in the transformation of cells, and actually measured the oxygen pressures inside tumors in the living body.

Dr Warburg did not physically interfere with the experimental healthy cells in any way, and he did not employ chemicals, heat or radiation—he merely reduced their supply of oxygen. When he reduced the oxygen needed by the cells for normal respiration by thirty-five per cent, they de-differentiated to become cancer cells.

How can cells in the human body with an unrestricted air supply be deprived of oxygen? Answer: toxemia (unhealthy blood).

Blood carries oxygen to the body's cells together with the nutrients the cells need to utilize the oxygen (the vitamins and minerals from which respiratory enzymes are made). Unhealthy blood is low both ways and sluggish in its flow. Dr Warburg's experiment in the laboratory took only days, but in real life cancer may take years, maybe few, maybe many, depending on the degree of toxemia, but when the critical point is reached the end result is the same.

Thus cancer, as with heart disease, can to a large extent be predicted just by observing a person's dietary and other living habits. A proper blood test which took into account blood viscosity and oxygen levels as well as the usual factors would be more precise. As previously explained, in conditions of toxemia before symptoms of impending disease become apparent, there appear in the blood microorganisms which increase in numbers as the *milieu interieur* further deteriorates. These are the pleomorphic microbes described in Chapter 5. The relationship between this indicator of toxemia and the subsequent incidence of cancer was observed in a study of twenty-five patients over a twenty-year period by Dr Guy Owens, a surgeon in Amarillo, Texas. He said in 1979:

"We selected 25 cases from my practise where the organism was repeatedly found during blood counts. They were run of the mill office cases, being male, female, old and young, but apparently in average good health. Over a 20 year period, 23 of these people came down with malignancy of one kind or another . . . proven by surgery and proper pathologic examination. Two cases were lost from our records although one was known to have died from an obscure abdominal condition."

It is easy to understand why researchers concentrating on studying one disease can easily be led to false conclusions having identified a microbe present at the scene, and why the cancer/virus controversy went on for years. However, Dr Owens knew that all people carry within them these organisms and that it was their multiplication and behavior that indicated a pathological condition. What he did not know was how the pathological condition caused normal body cells to change into cancer cells.

Differentiation and De-differentiation

In brief, the transformation of normal cells into abnormal (cancer) cells is a predictable, biological event, obeying natural biological laws in circumstances that give the cells no other choice if they are to survive individually. In Chapter 3 it was explained how in conditions of constipation, normal aerobic bacteria in the colon are forced to change into anaerobic bacteria. In a similar fashion, when body cells are deprived of oxygen or the enzymes necessary to utilize oxygen they will endeavor to survive by anaerobic means, and to do this they must change in form, ie, de-differentiate, to a more primitive form.

Differentiation is the process that takes place in a developing embryo during pregnancy by which primitive, unspecialized embryo cells, as they multiply, change in form to the different specialized cells required to form the different organs of the baby's body. At conception, when egg and sperm unite to form one cell which then subdivides and multiplies, the new cells—called embryonic cells—are all the same: they are primitive in form, largely anaerobic, and multiply rapidly without constraint. And although they are different to the mother's own body cells and therefore foreign to her body, because of what is known as "blocking factor" they are not challenged by her immune system.

When the embryo attaches to the mother's circulatory system and begins to receive nourishment and oxygen from the mother's blood, the embryonic cells become fully aerobic, ie dependent on oxygen. As the embryo continues to grow, the embryonic cells change in form: they become different from each other in order to construct the different organs of the new body, so that they are identifiable as bone cells, muscle cells, skin cells and so on. They are differentiated.

In understanding cancer, the points to remember are that embryo cells are initially primitive, undifferentiated, largely anaerobic and multiply without constraint, whereas fully differentiated, specialized cells in normal tissues are aerobic and their subdivision and growth is strictly constrained.

When bacteria, which are single primitive cell organisms, are deprived of oxygen they are capable of survival by reverting to the process of fermentation of nutrients in order to produce the energy they need. This process, called glycolysis, was the process used by primitive cells billions of years ago before oxygen became freely available in the sea and air, and is still part of the aerobic respiratory process employed by oxygen-using cells of living creatures today.

Glycolysis is an inefficient process which liberates only small amounts of energy from a given amount of blood sugar, leaving a residue of pyruvic acid which is converted to lactic acid and eliminated. Oxygen-using (aerobic) cells still retain glycolysis in the initial stages of their respiratory cycle but are immensely more efficient because they are capable of taking the pyruvic acid resultant from glycolysis and combining it with oxygen, which process not only liberates about fifteen times more energy but at the same time leaves only carbon dioxide and water as by-products, substances which are completely harmless and easily eliminated.

In order to survive by fermentation, aerobic bacteria must change into a more primitive form, and because fermentation is so inefficient, more fuel (blood sugar) must be consumed and a lot of acid produced. This process occurs in the mouth when the natural bacteria there are deprived of oxygen by food residues stuck between the teeth, and the acid so produced eats away the tooth enamel to make the cavities we call tooth decay. Similarly, aerobic bacteria normal in the colon (bowel) change into anaerobic bacteria when putrifying residues of protein and fat cause constipation and acids and other toxins are produced, many of which find their way into the bloodstream.

When lipotoxemia and acidic conditions of the blood result in deterioration of the lymph which sustains the tissue cells of the body, the cells may be deprived of oxygen or deprived of the enzymes they need to utilize oxygen. When this occurs the *milieu interieur*, polluted, is referred to as the cancer milieu.

Like bacteria (which are cells), the cells of the human body are similarly capable of reverting to a more primitive form when forced to by interference to their normal respiration, and the more their aerobic respiration is curtailed, the more primitive they must become in order to survive. Thus, for a normal fully differentiated cell, eg a lung cell, to change into a more primitive form it must de-differentiate, and in degrees lose its identity as a lung cell, and resemble more and more the primitive embryo cells from which the body originated. The degree of de-differentiation is proportional to the degree the cell is dependent on fermentation to survive, and when the cell reaches a certain stage of primitiveness it forgets its allegiance to the body as a whole and starts to reproduce as primitive cells do, heedless of the body's normal constraints. This unrestrained growth of increasingly de-differentiated cells is cancer, and the tumor at the site of origin is called the primary tumor.

The degree of de-differentiation determines the primitiveness of the cells and therefore their rate of growth, which means that the malignancy of the cancer is directly related to the degree of de-differentiation, fermentation and production of lactic acid. Thus the cancer growth proceeds in a vicious circle because the lactic acid and other waste products of the cancer cells worsen further the cancer milieu which started the process off in the first place. Moreover, because the cancer cells resemble embryonic cells in structure and function they are to some degree capable of producing the same blocking factor embryonic cells do, which inhibits the immune system from attacking them.

Metastasis—The Main Danger

Cells do not have to be fully de-differentiated to grow as cancer, and therefore pathology tests can usually identify them with the tissue of their origin. Thus, when cancer cells migrate in the blood and lymph and start secondary tumors elsewhere in the body (metastatis), the site of the primary growth can usually be determined by examination of cells from the secondary. The secondary growths are the most fast growing, because although at the tissue of their origin the normal constraints to growth still tend to control the primary cancer, away from the tissue of origin the constraints do not exist. Primary tumors therefore are usually slow growing, and it is only when metastasis occurs that cancer is considered to be terminal.

As the cancer growth proceeds, the process becomes a vicious circle in which more and more of the body's supply of blood sugar is squandered in the wasteful production of lactic acid and so the entire body, poisoned and starved of sustenance, wastes away in the condition known as cachexia.

Important—Note Well

When primary tumors liberate stray cancer cells into the circulation, for metastasis to occur such cells must first escape destruction by the immune system, and then lodge in a location where the circulation is blocked by a thrombus (fibrin clot). This was demonstrated by Dr Summer Wood of Boston in 1958 (AMA Archives of Pathology, Vol. 66, October 1958). About the same time, Dr L. Michaels of Canada reasoned that if no clots were allowed to form, then metastasis from a primary tumor could not occur, and that people with only primary cancers would in that case be in a much safer situation. This he proved to be the case. He studied the medical histories of a large number of heart and stroke patients kept on permanent anti-coagulant drug treatment to protect their blood circulation, to ascertain the incidence of cancer deaths among them, and found the incidence to be only one eighth of the expected number. The study covered the equivalent of 1569 patient/years and there was not a single case of death by cancer metastasis in the group. Thus it is easy to understand why fat is a major factor in most cancers and why herbal anti-coagulants such as garlic, aloe vera and so on assist people on high-fat diets to avoid cancer.

The major factor underlying the cancer process is improper diet. The incidence of all kinds of cancer is related more to the high intake of cooked food containing fat, protein, cholesterol, salt and preservatives than to anything else, although anything at all detrimental to the purity of the bloodstream must one way or another contribute to the problem. The deprivation of oxygen to the cells is caused not only by high blood viscosity, poor circulation and low oxygen levels, but also by the absence of the enzymes needed to process the oxygen. The respiratory enzymes may be absent because of nutrients missing from the diet[1], or the respiratory enzymes may be inhibited by carcinogens in the bloodstream derived from sources such as food, smoking, alcohol, putrefaction in the colon and poisons from infected teeth.

[1] See "Mineral Deficiencies" in Chapter 14, which outlines Dr Maynard Murray's prevention of cancer in mice.

Dr Joseph Issels of Germany, who has researched and treated cancer for fifty years, asserts that poisoning from infected teeth is one of the prime causes of cancer, and this viewpoint is supported by Dr Mulhim Hassan of Lebanon in his book *Prevention and Cure of Cancer.*

However, of all the many factors which in one way or another contribute to the deterioration of the *milieu interieur* and predispose the body to cancer, constipation appears to be by far the worst. It is important to remember that a regular daily bowel movement does not mean the absence of constipation; what counts is the time food residues take to transit the digestive tract. On the traditional Western diet of mainly cooked unsuitable food the transit time is about seventy-two hours, which means that "regular" or not, there are always stagnant putrefying residues occupying the colon producing carcinogenic substances, some of which provoke local problems and some of which perfuse back into the bloodstream. Sir William Arbuthnot Lane,[2] the famous British surgeon, repeatedly emphasized he had never known a single case of cancer that had not been preceded by prolonged intestinal stasis.

[2] Sir William Arbuthnot Lane, BART CB; Consulting Surgeon to Guys Hospital; Consulting Surgeon to The Hospital for Sick Children, London; President of The New Health Society; author of *The Prevention of the Diseases Peculiar to Civilization* (1929).

In his surgical practice, Sir William noted that so common were diseased colons he was forced to conclude the colon to be the seat of most chronic diseases, and for some time he specialized in the removal of diseased colons. This procedure confirmed his ideas because most of his patients' chronic disorders cleared up very quickly after losing their colons, and their overall health improved. Eventually he realized that the colon was not, itself, a troublesome organ, and became diseased only because of the kind of food people ate, and that the resulting disorders were the result of what he called 'auto-intoxication'. It was at this time in his career he became converted to the concept of natural health and thereafter concentrated his efforts on educating patients rather than cutting pieces out of them.

Professor Aviles of the Biochemistry of Cancer Department, Guadalajara, Mexico reported that out of 7715 cancer patients examined by him over a fifteen-year period, at least ninety-nine per cent had suffered from constipation and that the degree of malignancy was parallel to the degree of constipation. Doctors Dennis Burkitt and Hugh Trowell, who both spent twenty-five years working in rural Africa, agreed that in those areas where the diet of the natives consisted almost entirely of fruit and vegetables, the "transit time" of the natives was about twenty-four hours, there was no such thing as constipation and cancer was non-existent. Dr E. H. Tipper in his book *The Cradle of the World and Cancer* (1927) said:

> "Cancer has been suspected of being a disease of civilization. Judging from my experience in general practise in London, twenty years in West Africa, and again in rural England, I am convinced that this is true. It is due to the conventionalism and bad feeding of civilization, and is an exact index of the degree to which the alimentary tract has deviated from its natural and normal state of health. In the case of cancer, constipation and excessive meat-eating should be the two suspects, when they are present cancer is rife, where absent there is none."

However, despite the foregoing, a low-fat, low-cholesterol diet is no guarantee against cancer unless toxemia from other sources is avoided, and such toxemia is possible on a high-protein vegetarian diet containing excessive quantities of grain products and lentils. The author's observations of cancer occurring among conscientious followers of the Pritikin diet led him to suspect the heavy dependence on grain products, having previously noted the exacerbation of arthritis which accompanied excessive intake of these foods. These suspicions were confirmed by the results of the US Government's six-year Multiple Risk Factor Intervention Trial (MRFIT), evaluated in the *Journal of the American Medical Association* (*JAMA*) in Janunary 1987. The trial was conducted to evaluate the risk factors involved in coronary heart disease, in particular the relationship between blood cholesterol levels and heart attacks among the 12,000 male participants. As expected, the group with the lowest cholesterol levels (below 4.3) suffered only one quarter the death rate from heart attacks than the group with the highest cholesterol but, surprisingly, this low cholesterol group suffered just on fifty per cent more deaths from cancer than all the other groups (whose death rates from cancer were all about the same as each other), which led some doctors to believe that low cholesterol levels could actually favor the onset of cancer. But this did not make sense because all previous knowledge showed low cholesterol to be protective against cancer.

However, bearing in mind the acid-producing effects of excessive consumption of grains and other high-protein vegetables, we can explain the apparent anomaly. As Nathan Pritikin had already demonstrated before the MRFIT trial began, the only way to achieve such big reductions in blood cholesterol is to eliminate almost entirely from the diet all cholesterol containing foods and in their place substitute cholesterol-free foods such as grain products, lentils, vegetables and fruit. This diet works wonderfully to lower cholesterol and to improve circulation, but because too little fruit is eaten and because vegetables are eaten mostly cooked and are less satisfying, and because grain products and lentils are not limited and *are* satisfying, it is the grain products and lentils that are consumed in excessive quantities capable of producing acid toxemia, despite the fact constipation may no longer exist. Pritikin advised the intake of copious quantities of raw salad to offset the acid formed from the grains, but it's a fact that most people just don't like eating a lot of salad and would rather stuff themselves with rice, oats or spaghetti, all of them acid forming.

The cancer process, like atherosclerosis, may take many years to develop, and the onset of the cancer growth itself usually appears in middle age or later when the vital organs have degenerated to the stage they can no longer maintain a reasonable degree of purity of the *milieu interieur*. In the years preceding the appearance of cancer as a growth, the tissues pass through a stage known as pre-cancer, and while the body's immune system is capable of reasonable function, any cancer cells that form, at least in the early stages, may be quickly destroyed by the immune system's white cells, providing of course that the white cells are capable of reasonable function. It should be noted that fat and cholesterol in the blood severely inhibit the white cells' activity.

Dr Max Gerson, referring to experiments with animals, said that whatever chemical assault was necessary to cause cancer in them the cancer never commenced until after the liver function became impaired, "together with pathological changes in the kidneys, spleen and lymphatic apparatus". Gerson illustrated this point with an experiment in which he completely eliminated cancer in a rat simply by interconnecting its blood circulation with that of a healthy rat whose liver was fully functional.

Primary cancer occurs mainly in tissues which in their day-to-day function have a constant wearing out and renewal of cells: tissues such as the skin, the lining of the digestive tract, the respiratory tract and the female genital canal. Apart from the fact that the cells in these tissues tend to rapidly reproduce anyway, these tissues are exposed to irritation of various kinds which promotes normal renewal growth. New growth requires temporary de-differentiation of cells in any tissue, and if the tissue is in a pre-cancerous state any irritation or injury may be sufficient to trigger partially de-differentiated cells into becoming cancer cells. It has been postulated in the past that irritation or injury may be a cause of cancer, a postulation which of course in incorrect because irritation or injury cannot trigger cancer in healthy tissue.

Cancer is often also linked with emotional factors such as worry and grief. The two factors, physical injury and emotional stress, time and again precede the appearance of cancer, separately or together, and have often been thought to be primary causes of cancer. However, it is clear

Horne - 21st Century

diabetes - 67-68, 268-269
p92 - herbal anti coagulants eg garlic,
aloe vera, etc - helps avoid cancer

that cancer occurs only in tissue that is pre-cancerous beforehand and that irritation and emotional stress are only secondary factors, irritation by its effect on triggering cell growth, and emotional stress by its effect on depressing the cancer-fighting ability of the body's immune system. Probably in the same way emotional stress favors the onset of cancer, it has long been observed by physicians that people with melancholy personalities seem to be more prone to the disease, it being proposed there is such a thing as a "cancer personality". On the other hand, it would seem more likely that the melancholy disposition is not a cause of cancer but, like the cancer itself, just another symptom of a toxic bloodstream.

Hormone imbalance may also enter the picture; breast cancer is often associated with high levels of estrogen, the female growth hormone, and it should be noted that overproduction of estrogen is caused by high levels of fat in the diet. As Nathan Pritikin explained, it is the abnormal production of estrogen due to fat in the Western diet that accounts for the premature sexual development and bigger breasts of today's young girls.

Smoking is considered to be the primary cause of lung cancer, but research has shown that its role in producing lung cancer is mainly that of an irritant triggering new growth in tissue already pre-cancerous. Asbestos causes similar irritation. The role of smoking as a real primary cancer cause is its effect of introducing carbon monoxide into the bloodstream and reducing available oxygen to the tissues. Strong sunshine is thought to be the prime cause of skin cancer, but it is no such thing; it is an irritant which triggers new cell growth it is true, but skin cancer only eventuates in skin which is pre-cancerous, and when people adopt a low-fat, low-cholesterol diet they find the skin cancers no longer occur.

Billions and billions of dollars have been spent on desperate research to find a cure for cancer, a quest doomed to failure from the start even though doctors talk about various rates of cures obtained by surgery, radiation and chemotherapy. A person is regarded as cured of cancer if after the operation the cancer does not re-appear in five years, and all through that anxious five years or in the next maybe less anxious five years (if the patient lasts that long) nobody knows if and when the cancer will "strike" again.

Cancer can be considered "cured" only if the causes underlying it are understood and permanently removed, so that the affected tissue can become healthy again by the process of natural healing, called a spontaneous remission in medical parlance. The simple solution to the cancer problem is to stop doing the things that cause cancer.

At the meeting of Nobel Laureates in Lindau, Germany on 30 June 1966, Dr Otto Warburg concluded his address as follows:

> "Nobody today can say that one does not know what cancer and its prime cause be. On the contrary, there is no disease whose prime cause is better known, so that today ignorance is no excuse that one cannot do more about prevention. The prevention of cancer will come there is no doubt, for man wishes to survive. But how long prevention will be avoided depends on how long the prophets of agnosticism will succeed in inhibiting the application of scientific knowledge in the cancer field. In the meantime, millions of people must die of cancer unnecessarily."

Note: For additional hope and understanding of cancer *see* "Recommended Reading on Cancer" in the Appendix.

CHAPTER 13

Sexuality and Homosexuality

Sexual inadequacies and distortions take their inevitable toll in epidemic proportions: impotence, frigidity, pornography, masochism, sadism, promiscuity—and homosexuality.

Homosexuality, like these other manifestations of dis-ease, is a symptom of disturbed personality. Its origins lie in the same breeding grounds as those that stunt the maturation of so many heterosexuals.

Dr Robert Kronemeyer,
author of *Overcoming Homosexuality*
(Macmillan 1980)

In the spring a young man's fancy lightly turns to thoughts of love.

Alfred, Lord Tennyson (1809–1892)

Today it is different. As our society slips further and further away from Nature and people become more and more anxious about the future, they have become increasingly dependent all year round on the sensual "pleasures of the flesh" to fill a void in their lives which should not be there. Like health, happiness, love and contentment are the natural birthrights of all people but which, however, to a great extent we have been deprived of by our modern way of life. This deprivation is the void we attempt to fill by more or less artificial means. And as with using medicine to treat a physical disorder, all that this attempt yields is temporary relief until the effect of the medicine wears off.

Chasing sexual gratification in the attempt to fulfil the natural desire for romantic love and security (of which combination sex is an important component) is an act more of desperation than natural desire. Preoccupation with sex, like greed and corruption, is a sign of sickness in a population just as much as are the ever-increasing rates of other mental illnesses and other common diseases of degeneration.

A healthy appetite for sex is natural, but when pornography, violence and cacophonic noise begin to dominate our sources of entertainment, bringing us stress instead of happiness, and when these affronts to decency become accepted, even desirable, in society, then what we see is the beginning of a slide which will make the decline and fall of the Roman Empire look like a Sunday School picnic.

Over-sexuality is a form of neurosis, not a sign of vigor and health, and like homosexuality it is an abnormal condition which does not occur among any species of animals on Earth, including humans, when a natural environment prevails.

People often conjecture about the "purpose of life". Why are we here? It seems the main purpose of life is to ensure the continuation of the species, and for this reason every kind of living thing on earth, plant or animal, is abundantly endowed—over-endowed—with the capability of procreation. So nobody can say that a healthy sex appetite is unnatural. It is imperative in Nature that there is always an overproduction of individuals in any species in case of adverse circumstances which could threaten the survival of the species as a whole. If the individuals comprising the surplus are not needed and cannot be sustained in the prevailing circumstances, they simply die, but always the total remains as high as the circumstances of space and food supplies allow.

Plants have an advantage over animals in that if their survival is threatened they can produce seeds which can lie dormant for years if necessary until favorable circumstance return. Thus in drought conditions, grasses, weeds and other plants, sensing death by dehydration, will go prematurely to seed before dying of thirst. Animals of course have the advantage over plants in that they are mobile and can travel in search of water and food.

Fruit-growers, knowing these things about plants, realize that if conditions are too favorable for their fruit trees the trees won't trouble to produce as much fruit, so by manipulating the watering at the right time they induce stress to the trees to encourage them to produce more fruit. The tree does this to ensure there will be more seeds, and the farmer gets a better crop. Thus the urge to reproduce is increased in life-threatening situations.

What about animals? Stress influences the chemistry of the blood, the most well known of the various effects being that of the secretion of adrenalin to arouse the senses and increase the metabolic rate in threatening situations. Denied the chance of fighting or fleeing the threat of death, a "last-resort" animal instinct is that to reproduce. Sensing the imminence of death, cattle awaiting slaughter at abattoirs will become sexually aroused, while people awaiting death in the gas chambers in Nazi extermination camps in World War II would, in a similar fashion, indulge in sex.

Another illustration of abormal sexual activity is given in Louis Kuhne's *New Science of Healing* (1894):

"It is an old and well-known fact to farmers, that an unnaturally increased sexual impulse among cattle is a sure sign of a disease having broken out. And it is the same with man, as anyone can observe who will look about him. I need only mention here the abnormal sexual excitement on the part of consumptives.

Sexual impulse in healthy man is something altogether different from that unbridled lust we see so often today."

In situations in which animals are deprived of freedom and normal healthy activity, they will display sexual depravity along with brutality and other unnatural behavior they would never in their natural environment indulge in. Dr Solly Zuckerman was a distinguished professor of anatomy at Birmingham University in the 1920s and 30s, and in the study of humans and the other primates wrote a book from which it was intended humans could learn more about themselves. The book, *The Social Life of Monkeys and Apes* (1932), described various behavioral patterns of primates in captivity in the London Zoo but, as Robert Ardrey pointed out in his book *African Genesis* (1961), conclusions drawn from behavior in captivity are not representative of an animal's true instinct in nature:

> "The famous anatomist cannot be blamed for presuming that the sex-obsessed activities of London baboons reflected true primate behavior, or for drawing the logical conclusion that the powerful magnet of sexual attraction must be the force that holds primate societies together. But over and over we shall encounter in this narrative the disastrous consequences of applying utter logic to a false premise. [Which goes to show that doctors are not the only people who jump to wrong conclusions by applying logic to a false premise.] And Zuckerman's premise was false. The creature whom we watch in the zoo is one denied by the conditions of his captivity the normal flow of his instinctual energies. Neither the drives of hunger nor the fear of the predator stir the idleness of his hours. Neither the commands of normal society nor the demands of territorial defence pre-empt the energies with which Nature has endowed him. If he seems a creature obsessed with sex, then it is simply because sex is the only instinct for which captivity permits him an outlet."

Desmond Morris has pointed out that to call a city an "asphalt jungle" is totally wrong because it is much more like a "human zoo", in which zoo flourishes crime, homosexuality, rape and obsession with food, drink and sex. Nor outside of cities are humans free and natural either, but they are freer and closer to Nature than their city counterparts and are blessed accordingly. It is clear that the further a community is distanced from an unnatural environment and the closer it conforms to Nature, the better is the likelihood its inhabitants will resemble true and proper human beings.

The fact that the majority of people prefer to live in cities demonstrates the natural instinct in humans to congregate, for mental stimulus and other advantages, but in man's primitive evolutionary past high density living was not possible and the appetite for carnivals and excitement had to be satisfied by the annual tribal get-togethers like the corroborees of Aboriginals or the sing-sings in the New Guinea highlands. Cities are man-made traps as much as are alcohol, cigarettes, junk food, medicine and pollution, and to those who are aware of the pitfalls they need present no great hazard.

The ways of Nature, mysterious and exact, are always directed at restoring homeostasis, not only within the body but within whole population groups. If for instance in a community of bees of a certain hive a greater than usual proportion of worker bees is lost due to bushfire or some other reason, or if a lot of soldier bees are killed defending the hive from predatory ants, straight away the output of eggs by the queen bee is altered to produce a higher proportion of either worker bees or soldier bees as the situation requires to restore the correct balance in the hive's population. In human populations, the death rate among males is slightly higher than among females, and this is compensated for by a similar slightly higher proportion of male children born than female. What mysterious natural force controls this ratio? Is this ratio variable should there be a change for some reason in danger factors among humans?

One factor associated with aggressiveness and oversexuality is the high consumption of meat in the diet, and when people give up eating meat to become vegetarian they report that their natures become more placid and less sexually aggressive. Statistics show that vegetarians, generally, have a far better life expectancy than meat-eaters, and therefore it is a reasonable supposition that vegetarians feel less urgency to reproduce. The self-regulating mechanism within all living things to increase the reproductive urge when survival is threatened works, it seems, not only to increase the urge in humans who eat a lot of meat, but takes into account also that the wastage rate among male meat-eaters is greater than that among females. Statistics can be used to prove anything so they say; what do you make of this one? A 1987 report from official British statistics stated that in 1980–82, for every 100 girls fathered by butchers and meat-cutters there were 121 boys, compared with the national average of 105.6 boys for every 100 girls. This fact, in light of how Nature works to preserve balance, would seem to confirm that meat-eating is a hazard, and in the further light of the fact that meat-eating tends to excite sexual arousal more than does vegetarianism, thus is provided another example of how "living dangerously" leads to sexual excesses.

For what it's worth, a recent article in Brisbane's *The Courier Mail* asserted that a woman could plan to influence the sex of her future child by means of diet. It said that if a woman's diet (obviously for some time before conception) included lots of lettuce, watercress, broccoli, asparagus, radishes, cucumber, cabbage and cauliflowers she would have a great chance of having a girl. And if she ate lots of ham, bacon, smoked salmon, salty mineral water, dried beans and broad beans, she would have "a sterling" chance of producing a boy. Whether butchers ever marry vegetarians the author has no idea.

Thus it should never be assumed that what appear to be peculiar quirks of Nature are simply random errors. Not at all; they are predictable consequences of abnormal circumstances, more often than not man-made.

Homosexuality

Recently, in calling for a change in laws regarding homosexuals, a group of more than forty psychologists in Queensland agreed that the latest research showed that homosexuals made up a large proportion of the population and that homosexuality was quite natural.

But it is absurd to conclude that homosexuality is quite natural simply because a large proportion of the population is comprised of homosexuals. That the diseases of civilization are all natural consequences of an unnatural lifestyle doesn't mean we should regard the diseases as natural. Cancer, heart disease and the other diseases of civilization do not occur in animals living in Nature, but they often do in domesticated animals. The only thing natural about them is that they occur as a natural reaction to unnatural circumstances. Homosexuality is a disorder not in accord with Nature and, like cancer, heart disease or neurosis, is a reaction to circumstances non-existent in Nature but common in man-made circumstances.

In calling for recognition that homosexuality is natural, the panel of psychologists at the same time referred to three different studies in which the rates of attempted suicide of young homosexuals were reported as twenty per cent, eighteen per cent and twenty-one per cent respectively. The reports did not reveal how many of the suicide attempts succeeded, but whereas the psychologists presumed the attempts resulted from the despair of non-acceptance in society by an otherwise normal person, to other psychologists the same facts indicate an underlying personality disorder, which disorder in the first place is the reason for homosexuality.

The tendency to regard homosexuality as more or less normal is influenced by data from the Kinsey Report on sexual behavior, which gave the impression that almost everybody has within them the potential to become homosexual in circumstances which deprive them of contact with the opposite sex. That such segregation as in prisons and boarding schools, etc, results in homosexual behavior is well known, but the Kinsey data showed that only about one third of jail prisoners indulged in such behavior and that no heterosexual prisoner continued with homosexual relations once they became free. Homosexuals, however, are people who at no time are sexually attracted to the opposite sex, even finding the opposite sex sexually repugnant, but instead have a powerful and constant desire for sexual relations with people of their own sex.

An argument used to demonstrate that homosexuality is natural is that male animals are commonly observed to mount each other and appear to perform sexually, but whether they achieve satisfaction or not does not denote homosexuality, because homosexuality means complete aversion to sexual relations with the opposite sex and complete sexual desire for one's own sex, a situation which does not occur in Nature among dogs or any other animals.

The Kinsey data concluded that in the USA one person in every ten was a homosexual, and this proportion has been, by rule of thumb, accepted to be pretty much the same in all populations. But other studies have shown otherwise. Whereas history records the existence of homosexuality as far back as history goes, and records the homosexual behavior of emperors, kings, queens, scholars and scientists over the centuries, there are also records showing that in some remote and more primitive populations homosexuality is unknown, while in other population groups it occurs in widely varying degrees. That the highest incidence of homosexuality coincides with the general level of stressful influences in a community and that the lowest incidence coincides with the degree of happiness and health in remote and unstressed populations indicates that, like many conditions of physical disease, it is just as unnatural as the mental breakdowns, depression and neuroses so common in civilization.

Studies of primitive natives reveal that while in some populations homosexuality is non-existent or rare, in other populations it is fairly common; but the same pattern still holds—among the placid, happy, untroubled people homosexuality did not occur, while among fighting tribes and headhunters it did.

Dr Robert Kronemeyer of New York, after twenty-five years of clinical experience helping homosexual men and women, wrote a book, *Overcoming Homosexuality* (Macmillan, 1980). In this book Dr Kronemeyer related the observations of Dr Margaret Mead, who earlier this century studied the behavior of many native groups of the South Seas. Describing the people of Samoa, Dr Mead called them "peaceful and constructive . . . a people who plant and reap, fish and build, feast and dance in a world where no one is hurried . . . and life is harmonious and uninhibited". Babies were breastfed generously, and "children are loved and cared for and reared in large stable families that do not rely on some tenuous tie between two parents for their own security". Dr Mead noted the only homosexuality observed among the Samoans was the casual relationships between adolescent boys which they soon outgrew.

Other healthy populations in which homosexuality was never known were the Comanche Indians, and the Hunzas. It is significant that, as reported by Dr McCarrison, in nine years he worked in Hunza he observed not one case of cancer or heart disease either.

"Informed opinion" of psychologists agrees that sexual orientation is developed in early childhood and that, once formed, homosexuality is not amenable to clinical intervention. One psychologist stated that research showed homosexuality was not an unnatural or psychiatric disorder, that it was like being left- or right-handed, and that no amount of intervention can change it. But hold on for a minute—not long ago heart disease was said to be irreversible, cancer was considered always fatal and today so too is AIDS. But as we have seen, these opinions were wrong. Just as epidemiological studies of heart disease and cancer have revealed the underlying causes of these illnesses, the same kind of studies reveal the factors underlying homosexuality; and the fact that homosexuality is an effect produced by unnatural human factors means that homosexuality is not natural in humans at all, but is an aberration which need not occur.

A study of 1500 San Francisco gays by the Institute for Sex Research in 1978 concluded that homosexuality in itself is not abnormal and that most homosexuals are not dissatisfied with their lives; most of them are "stable, happy, and well adjusted". Twenty per cent of the men said they had attempted suicide and about half of them each admitted to having had at least 500 sexual partners. Does this indicate happiness and adjustment? Having seen the movie *Word is Out*, produced by homosexuals about homosexuals, social commentator Harriett Van Horne wrote in her syndicated column: "Their stories are mostly very sad . . . By any standard, most are lost, lonely, sick, and altogether heart-breaking . . . Whatever possessed these people to call homosexuals 'gay'?"

Studies have shown the single factor shared invariably by all homosexuals, male and female, is an unhappy childhood which in most cases commenced with an incomplete mother/child relationship, and was perhaps further degraded by parental discord and feelings of insecurity. In view of this fact, the findings of a recent report are not surprising. The British research body "One plus One", in its report "Marital Breakdown", stated that the children of divorced parents were twice as likely to display delinquent behavior, four times as likely to suffer stomach ulcers or colitis before age twenty-six, were more accident prone, troubled, drifting, underachieving, and as adults far more prone to psychiatric illness and drinking problems.

"Homosexuals are made, not born 'that way' ", said Dr Kronemeyer, "from my twenty-five years' experience as a clinical psychologist, I firmly believe that homosexuality is a learned response to early painful experiences and that it can be *unlearned*. For these homosexuals who are unhappy with their life and find effective therapy, it is 'curable'."

So many factors affect a person's prospect for health and happiness, however, it is foolish to try and blame perhaps only one or two for any particular upset. A person's prospects for the future begin with the parents' health before they are even conceived. Most crucial is the diet and behavior of the mother while she is pregnant, and after birth breastfeeding and loving care and training continue the influence which will determine the wellbeing or otherwise of the future adult. It is common knowledge that the effects of emotional stress, poor diet, alcohol and smoking on a pregnant woman have consequential adverse effects on the baby she is carrying, effects such as physical deformities and mental retardation in varying degrees. That drugs, either "recreational" or medical, have similar effects, in some cases very severe, is also well known. Therefore it is quite possible that tendency towards homosexuality may be acquired to some extent congenitally as was demonstrated by Dr Francis Pottenger's dietary experiments with animals at San Diego in the 1940s (see pp. 18 and 211).

In his book *The Wonderful World Within You* (1987), Dr Roger J. Williams described abnormalities in children that commonly occur due to dietary deficiencies experienced by mothers in pregnancy and by children in early life. Speaking of deficiencies of pantothenic acid and folic acid, which are only two nutrients out of many, he says that a deficiency of them alone may cause all sorts of deformities including malformation of hormone-producing glands. "When we realize", he said, "that these two relatively unfamiliar vitamins are essential to reproduction in animals and that deficiencies in these may produce serious deformities, we are led to wonder if deficiencies in human prenatal and postnatal nutrition may not also be responsible for many unexplained defects and deformities."

A recent study tending to support this view showed that there are biological differences between adult homosexuals and heterosexuals. The study, by neurologist Simon Le Vay at the Salk Institute for Biological Studies, San Diego, California, found that the hypothalamus—the part of the male brain governing sexual urges—is much smaller in homosexuals than in heterosexuals, and typically resembled a woman's rather than a heterosexual man's. Le Vay said: "I don't think this tells us the answer to the question 'are you born gay', but it does tell us that the topic of human sexuality can be studied biologically. Up to now it's been pretty much left to psychology."

The Spada Report, a survey of male homosexuality (James Spada 1979) described a study by F. J. Kellman of 85 homosexuals who had twin siblings. He found that among the 45 pairs in the survey who were fraternal twins, the incidence of homosexuality was about the same as between ordinary brothers and sisters, ie rarely were both homosexual. Among the 40 identical twins (those with the same genetic makeup), invariably both twins were homosexual, ie the incidence was 100%. These findings tend to indicate (but not prove) that it may well be that people are born gay.

Significant findings at the Brigham Young University in the USA indicate that stress during pregnancy can result in homosexual offspring. Dr D. E. Fleming and Dr R. W. Rhees, in experiments, subjected pregnant rats to psychological, nutritional and hormonal stress and then measured the behavioral characteristics of their male offspring. The results were compared to "normal" offspring of unstressed rats. "We found demasculinization and feminization tendencies," reported Dr Fleming. "Demasculinization, in that the test rats were not as active sexually in the male role; feminization was found where the males exhibited female-type behavior when placed with other males who were sexually aggressive. We are exploring possibilities that may have relevance to humans." The researchers observed that a definite correlation exists between the endocrinal systems of rats and humans. The predisposition towards homosexuality of male rats of the stressed mothers occurs because when the mother is under stress her body produces hormones that suppress production of androgen, necessary for the development of maleness in a male, although the male physical make-up appears normal. This occurs in the critical third trimester of the development of the fetus. The defect can be corrected by environmental influences—feminized male rats, when placed for long periods of time with females, will begin to exhibit normal male behavior. Three groups of mother rats were each subjected to a different form of stress, and in each group fifty per cent of the male offspring were affected.

One way or another, homosexuality is not a chosen way of life, and to quote Dr Kronemeyer again:

> "Homosexuality is a symptom of neurosis and of a grievous personality disorder. It is an outgrowth of deeply rooted emotional deprivations and disturbances that had their origins in infancy. It is manifested, all too often, by compulsive and self-destructive behavior that is the very antithesis of fulfilment and happiness. Buried under the 'gay' exterior of the homosexual is the hurt and rage that crippled his or her capacity for true maturation, for healthy growth and love.
>
> If I insist that homosexuality—the exclusive or predominant preference for same-gender sex relations for orgasmic satisfaction—is symptomatic of a psychic disorientation, I hasten to point out that I do not consider it any different, except possibly in the degree of pathology, from other neurotic manifestations of many heterosexuals . . .
>
> The earliest psychologists—Sigmund Freud, Richard von Krafft-Ebing, Havelock Ellis—were in agreement that homosexuality is a psychological malfunction that should be treated with tolerance and compassion. They might have disagreed on its cause, but they concurred that it was neither a crime nor a sin."

Conclusion

What is natural and what is unnatural? Rats kept in crowded captivity and fed on laboratory 'balanced' food display most unnatural behavior, they are nervous and agitated, they fight, they kill and eat their own young. Cats, confined in pens and fed pasteurized milk, lost condition and agility and their next generation was depleted by stillbirth, miscarriage and spontaneous abortion, with the survivors displaying many physical defects—neurosis and other abnormalities such as less anatomical differences between the sexes and homosexuality.[1] Similar defects occurred among zoo animals (Philadelphia Zoo) fed leftovers from restaurants, etc, which defects cleared after the animals' diets were changed to natural raw food.

What do captive zoo animals fed on defective diets have in common with humans? Zoologist Desmond Morris, introducing his book *The Human Zoo* (McGraw-Hill, 1969), had this to say:

"Under normal conditions, in their natural habitats, wild animals do not mutilate themselves, masturbate, attack their offspring, develop stomach ulcers, become fetishists, suffer from obesity, form homosexual pair-bonds, or commit murder . . .

The zoo animals in a cage exhibits all these abnormalities that we know so well from our human comparisons. Clearly, then, the city is not a concrete jungle, it is a human zoo . . .

Trapped, not by a zoo collector, but by his own brainy brilliance, he has set himself up in a huge, restless menagerie where he is in constant danger of cracking under the strain."

We have already discussed the deplorable health and moral standards of supposedly normal humans and how diet, liquor, nicotine and other drugs can cause mental and physical defects in their offspring. It is not a far-fetched notion then that a tendency towards homosexuality could already exist in a newborn child of a mother stressed and

[1] *The Effect of Heat Processed Foods and Pasteurized Vitamin D Milk on the Dentofacial Structures of Experimental Animals*, Dr Francis Pottenger, 1946, and *Disease in Captive Wild Animals and Birds*, Dr H. Fox, 1923.

not in the best of health herself, and that factors in childhood and adolescence tilt the balance one way or the other or perhaps result in a bisexual personality.

Be that as it may, let us take further advice from Dr Kronemeyer:

> "We would do well to bear in mind that effects indeed have causes and that 'there but for the grace of God go I . . .'
>
> Because it is a disabling neurosis, homosexuality merits an attitude of sympathy and understanding. Common decency prohibits us from discriminating against people who stammer or are hard of hearing or have birthmarks. To be biased against gays is comparably indecent—and absurd. Public and private strictures against homosexuals should be protested in the strongest terms. No burden of deportment, capability or reliability should be placed on homosexuals greater than that imposed on any other person. *As with all other disaffections, society should concern itself with increasing its awareness of the cause of homosexuality and the ways to prevention and 'cure'.*"

CHAPTER 14

Dieting for Health and Longevity

The Art of Living consists of dying young, but as late as possible.

Anon.

Dieting for health and dieting for longevity are not necessarily the same thing. Whereas dieting for immediate health improvement is of course worthwhile, a diet which may accomplish this in the short term may not necessarily be good enough to get the best long-term results. Dieting for longevity therefore must not only provide all the body's present requirements for good health, but do so with the least amount of strain on the vital organs in order to avoid as long as possible the degeneration we call old age.

The health of the body is only as good as the health, collectively, of all the body's individual cells. In turn, the health of the cells is determined by the quality of the lymph fluid that bathes them, ie the *milieu interieur*, which again is dependent on the purity of the bloodstream. Toxemia is the enemy.

So while it has long been a medical dictum that "a man is as old as his arteries", it is equally true that "a man is as healthy as his blood".

The composition of the blood is very complex and is maintained by the combined actions of all the vital organs. From the point of view of nutrition, it is the liver which takes in the products of digested food and redistributes them into the bloodstream to suit the rest of the body's requirements. And it is the liver and kidneys which receive back, also via the blood, the waste products of all the cells from which they sort out what components can be used again and what must be thrown out in the urine. For the maintenance of correct blood sugar levels, the liver depends on information from the pancreas, a dual purpose organ which not only secretes the insulin and glucogen used in the control of blood sugar but secretes, as an entirely separate function, the primary digestive enzyme juices used in the digestion of food. In the beginning and in the end, the status of health is determined almost entirely by the quality of the diet, because it is from the materials available in the diet that the liver constructs and orchestrates the entire spectrum of chemical processes upon which life depends. The design of the system is perfect; it is the quality of the diet that lets it down.

The Natural Diet of Man

Towards the end of World War II when the Americans invaded the Philippines and recaptured them from the Japanese, a lone Japanese soldier ran off into the jungle there and hid, firmly believing that sooner or later the tide of battle would turn again and Japan would in the end be victorious. He therefore decided to wait things out in the jungle. He waited twenty-five years, all the while avoiding human contact, and then one day emerged from the jungle and surrendered.

Returned to Japan and medically examined, the soldier amazed everybody—he looked so young compared to other middle-aged Japanese men. His teeth were perfect and his eyesight too. He displayed none of the usual signs of degenerative disease considered normal in civilization. And yet his life had not been easy. The only possible explanation for his physical preservation was that his diet for those years had been fruit, berries and various plants eaten raw, a diet similar to that of other wild primates and that of early humans before the discovery of fire.

Life of all kinds is most prolific in tropical regions both on land and sea, and this is not to be wondered at because it is in warm and moist conditions that enzymes work most efficiently. In such a warm, moist environment it is thought that life first appeared on Earth, and it is generally accepted that it was in the tropics that the early primates evolved from lower forms of life, to be followed by the evolution of the apes and then by the first humans.

In the plant kingdom, fruit trees were late arrivals on the evolutionary scene and it is highly probable that both fruit-bearing trees and the primates evolved concurrently, which accounts for the development in the primates of stereoscopic color vision, grasping hands, specialized teeth and jaw structure, appetite for sweet-tasting food, medium-length digestive tract, and so on. In their symbionic relationship, the fruit trees provided the primates with food and the primates unknowingly spread the fruit seeds wherever they ate or defecated, so ensuring the continued survival of the trees.

The study of comparative anatomy and the different natural diets of animals in the wild indicates strongly that the natural diet of early humans consisted predominantly of sweet fruits, and that even though millions of years have passed, the anatomy and digestive apparatus of humans has not changed and is therefore still best suited to fruit as the most suitable food. That this opinion is not just idle speculation can be quickly proven by any sick person who can break the addiction to our modern taste-stimulating foods and go on a diet of good quality fruit for just a few days. Of course the human digestive system is quite capable of handling foods of animal origin, including animal fats, but in only very limited amounts can it do so without strain, even when the foods are eaten raw as intended by Nature.

Thus it can be surmised that the ideal diet for man is one mainly of sweet fruits supplemented by various berries, green nuts, shoots and occasionally small amounts of foods of animal origin, all eaten raw. This is the sort of food eaten by man's closest relatives in Nature, the orangoutang and chimpanzee, both of which have an anatomy and digestive system almost identical to man's. Neither of these animals in the wild display tooth decay or any of the other diseases common to humans, but soon do so if kept in captivity and fed cooked and processed food.

If this surmise is correct, and if indeed humans can live in better health and for a longer time on such a natural diet, why ever did they change?

There is not a race of people anywhere today who, as a general rule, eat uncooked natural food; the majority of the world's populations base their diets on cooked grains of some kind or other, and the rest base theirs on cooked animal products supplemented by grain, dairy products and vegetables, all cooked. Fruit is looked upon more as a mere accessory to the various traditional diets rather than a sustaining food. How and why did this change come about?

Early man lived in small groups and, before the use of fire, ate his food raw like all the other creatures on Earth have done since life first began, their senses of sight, smell and taste indicating to them the foods most suitable to their systems. Population numbers were restricted by the amount of food available growing wild, but eventually with the discovery of fire it was found that various foods consumed by other animals but which were distasteful to the human palate could be made more edible by cooking, and more tasteful by artificially flavoring them with herbs and salt.

By the use of these new sources of food, greater populations could be supported, not only in areas already occupied, but in territory where food naturally suited for humans was not available.

As population pressures forced surplus people to move into less hospitable territory outside the tropics, they of necessity became reliant on a different diet, and on fire and primitive clothing for warmth. Sickness, when it occurred, was thought to be the work of evil spirits, and so witchdoctors had to be invented.

Greater challenges in a less benevolent environment led to continued brain development, and so it was in the temperate climatic zones of the world that technology commenced, leading to the advent of farming and the development of cereal crops from wild grasses. Continued competition for territory made warfare inevitable and this led again to greater technological development and so on. From all these changes a new breed of man emerged—one who had become "civilized" and had left his natural environment forever.

Next to the discovery of fire, the development of grain crops was the greatest factor leading to the human population explosion of today. Grain could be produced easily and, being storable, provided food for all seasons. More and more forest land was destroyed to grow crops and to make pasture to raise cattle, and according to their circumstances some populations came to base their diets on meat and dairy products and others based theirs on rice or wheat or other sorts of grain.

None of these diets provide ideal nutrition, and as civilization "progresses" and food becomes more and more preserved, processed, cooked and generally less and less natural, so humans everywhere display more signs of disease earlier and earlier in life. Even primitive races have always had their medicine men to protect their people from evil spirits and disease, but in civilization the superstition of medicine has got out of hand; "scientific medicine" has become a powerful industry consuming a vast amount of the national economy. But while the wild animals remain sleek and healthy without medicine, humans spend more and more money on "health care" and all the while just get sicker and sicker.

So illness can be seen to be a human phenomenon for which there are two main causes:

1 The use of unsuitable foods.
2 The cooking habit necessary to render unsuitable foods edible.

The unsuitability of our traditional Western diet has been explained in Chapter 2, but it may be asked why do people on other diets fare no better than us? Well, a few isolated populations such as the Hunzas do, but by and large the majority of other races are too heavily dependent on grains of some kind as the staple of their diets and grains are even less suitable to the human system than flesh foods.

Grain products (cereals) have been hailed as a health food by "victims" of the Western diet because they are low in fat, contain no cholesterol, are high in complex carbohydrate (starch) and high in fiber, the constipation fixer. Thus, switching to grains from the Western diet produces immediate benefits, but other problems soon arise. Grain products, supplying mainly starch, place a great burden on the digestive system. When mature, grains contain enzyme inhibitors which prevent digestion, but they are digestible when green (like sweet corn) or when cooked or after they have germinated. Grain-eating birds are equipped with crops in which grains, swallowed whole, germinate, whereupon the grains become digestible. Grains are indigestible raw, but even cooked, the complex carbohydrate requires great digestive effort to break down, and this is demonstrated by the fact that people of Eastern races, dependent on rice, develop a pancreas double its normal size and other signs of strain such as stunted intestinal villi. And unless rice (and other grains) are accompanied by liberal amounts of fresh vegetables and fruit in the diet, nutritional deficiencies occur and, at the same time, toxemia and acidosis capable of producing skin problems, arthritis, hardened arteries and cancer. That is why Orientals are generally smaller in stature and live no longer than Westerners.

Mineral Deficiencies

A less common and less suspected cause of disease is the deficiency (and sometimes excess) of minerals (trace elements) in food. Essential minerals are needed by the body to make enzymes, hormones, bone tissue, etc. Deficiencies usually occur because one or more trace minerals may be lacking in the soil in which the food plant was grown. Crops which are grown in deficient soil display poor condition and are susceptible to disease and attacks by pests.

Animals are more prone to display signs of mineral deficiencies than humans because humans consume food usually imported from all over the place whereas animals graze in the same areas all the time. There are some more or less isolated areas where people are dependent on crops grown in deficient soil such as in certain areas of Europe where iodine is lacking, the sign of which is the proneness of people to goitre. However, the subtleness of biochemistry is demonstrated by the fact that in Tasmania in 1949 it was noted that in some districts where iodine was plentiful in the soil there was, notwithstanding, a very high incidence of goitre which when iodine tablets were given only got worse. It turned out that the goitres were caused by an anti-thyroid factor contained in the milk of cows which were fed on marrow stem kale. White clover and cabbage under certain conditions of cultivation also sometimes contain an anti-thyroid factor capable of causing goitre. However, experiments at the Central Veterinary Laboratory in Weybridge, England, showed that marrow stem kale did not always contain the anti-thyroid factor which varied with the soil in which it was grown and the climatic conditions as well.

Thus it can easily be accepted that all other things aside, mineral imbalance alone in an otherwise healthy diet can severely impair the body's homeostasis, leading to symptoms of all kinds or the exacerbation of existing symptoms.

In the book *Soil Grass and Cancer* by Andre Voisin (Crosby Lockwood, London, 1959), from which the foregoing information was taken, the author described the functions of the various trace minerals in normal metabolism and the operation of the immune system, in particular the role of magnesium, copper and zinc in the functioning of the immune system.

Voisin emphasised that administering mineral salts to experimental animals led to wrong conclusions being formed because the only way the body can property assimilate minerals is in organic form, having been first taken up from the soil and changed to a colloid form by the plant used as food.

That the content of various minerals in a plant can vary enormously depending on the soil, the water content of the soil, the weather and so on means that the best way to obtain your minerals is from a variety of fresh, raw fruits and vegetables. Apart from vitamins and other nutrients in raw fruit and vegetables—preferably organically grown—the abundance of organic minerals they contain explains why patients with cancer respond so well when restricted to these foods.

That the mineral content of seawater is practically the same as blood is significant, and it is a fact, according to Dr Maynard Murray, that seawater contains all the trace minerals needed by humans. Dr Murray demonstrated forcefully that animals fed on his crops fertilized sparingly with diluted seawater exhibited superior growth and health compared to other animals. This is described in Dr Murray's book *Sea Energy Agriculture* (see page 91). Said Dr Murray:

> "The disease resistance of plants and animals in the sea is remarkably different from disease resistance in land animals and comparisons between animals of the same or similar species are most interesting. For example, fresh-water trout all develop terminal cancer of the liver at the average age of 5½ years; cancer has never been found in sea trout. It is also known that all land animals develop arterio-sclerosis, yet sea animals have never been diagnosed as arteriosclerotic. Investigators have also established the startling absence of disease in the sea, citing not only the absence of 'chronic' disease forms, but especially the general vigorous health of sea animals that has apparently lengthened life many times in comparison to similar land species.

These longevity differences are especially evident in such sea mammals as whales, seals and porpoises who have identical physiological systems with the majority of land animals important to man. And the major differences between sea and land life appear to be attributable to the superior food chain of the sea!''

Dr Murray's many experiments with all kinds of crops and animals all showed dramatic benefits from sea minerals. For instance:

"Started feeding mice both experimental and control, food that was raised on the Ray Heine and Sons Farm. The experimental food had been raised on soil fertilized with 2200 pounds (per acre) complete sea solids. The control food was the same as the experimental with the exception that it was not fertilized with complete sea solids. The food consisted of a combination of one part soybean, two parts oats, four parts corn, balanced food proteins, carbohydrates and fats for mammals.

C_3H mice were obtained for this feeding experiment. This strain of mice has been bred so all the females develop breast cancer which causes their demise. The mice were two months of age when received and started on the feeding experiments. The life expectancy of this strain for females is no more than nine months which included the production of two or three litters. The experimental and control groups both consisted of 200 C_3H mice and those fed on control food were all dead within eight months seven days. The experimental mice that were fed food grown on the sea solids fertilized soil lived until they were sacrificed at 16 months; definitive examination revealed no cancerous tissue. The experimental group produced ten litters compared to the usual two to three litters and none developed breast cancer.

In the next experiments, twenty-four rabbits

were obtained. Twelve were designated experimental and fed on food grown on sea solids while the remaining twelve were labelled control and fed accordingly. All of the rabbits were given a high cholesterol diet for six months which produces hardening of the arteries. The control group did develop hardening of the arteries and all had died within ten months. The experimental group did not exhibit hardening of the arteries.''

Another way people can obtain all the colloidal minerals they need is from fresh seawater taken about a teaspoon a day. *Health from the Sea and Soil*, by Charles B. Ahlson (Exposition Press, NY, 1962), described the remarkable health improvements by people with different ailments gained simply by taking fresh seawater. It is important that the seawater is fresh and unheated, because once heated the minerals lose their colloidal status necessary for the body to properly utilize them.

Fresh kelp and even dehydrated kelp is a good source of minerals from the sea and it is becoming common practice for farmers desiring the best crops while at the same time avoiding poisonous spraying to fertilize them with fertilizers derived from sea kelp.

And finally, on the subject of seawater minerals is a recent item from the *Queensland Fruit and Vegetable News*:

"There may be hope for Australian deserts if recent Israeli research is any indication.

Today thirsty plants are not only drinking but thriving on seawater at an experimental farm near the town of Ashkelon on the Mediterranean Sea.

Dr Dov Pasternak from the Boyko Institute at Ben Gurion University, is overseeing the project which is studying 150 species of plants irrigated by sea water.

The research into seawater for irrigation is directly related to the successful efforts of Dr Samuel Mendlinger, also from the Boyko Institute, to produce a special strain of sweet, high quality autumn melon grown on brackish water using drip and sprinkler irrigation.

Among other fruits and vegetables being successfully irrigated by saline water from underground aquifers are asparagus, broccoli, sorghum, olives, peas, and pomegranates.

Agricultural production in 14 southern Israel settlements is now based on underground saline water, and instead of costly desalination Israelis are taking advantage of Nature's abundance, learning to harness sea and sub-soil water to grow crops.''

The Pros and Cons of Cooking

All that cooking is good for is that it enables people to utilize grains for food and it renders other unsuitable foods such as meat and potatoes palatable and edible. Thus cooking enables a lot of people to sustain themselves on the only foods available to them, but there is a penalty to pay.

Reference has already been made in previous chapter to the problems encountered by eating cooked food. And the subject has been explained in depth in the author's previous books, *The Health Revolution* and *Improving on Pritikin*. In brief, the natural digestive process utilizes enzymes existing in raw food which, when the food is eaten, perform a considerable amount of predigestion (breaking down the food) in the upper cardiac section of the stomach before the main digestive system gets to work on it. Thus a great load is relieved from the pancreas, the organ that produces the main supply of digestive juices.

This natural benefit is entirely missing when cooked food is consumed because cooking destroys enzymes and, not only that, the pancreas is doubly penalized because of the difficult nature of the sort of food anyway when compared to the natural food man's system is designed for. Thus, as described by Dr Edward Howell in his books *The*

Status of Food Enzymes in Digestion and Metabolism (1946) and *Enzyme Nutrition* (1983), the human pancreas is invariably hypertrophied and twice its proper size compared with the relative sizes of those in wild animals and is accompanied by changes in the gonads, adrenals, pituitary and other ductless glands. Another adverse effect of cooking is that it renders minerals in the food less assimilable, while when cooking water is poured down the sink some of the minerals are lost altogether.

There is an association between the cooking and processing of food and the incidence of all diseases including cancer, and as proven in the sanatoria around the world, the best recoveries from chronic, so-called incurable diseases are made on diets composed of raw fruits and vegetables. This shows that when vital organs are at their lowest stage of function only such a diet makes it possible for them to provide the proper body chemistry to maintain health. That being the case, so must raw food provide the maximum benefit to anybody whether sick or well.

The Pros and Cons of Raw Food

First, the cons. The traditional foods to which we are accustomed are mostly inedible when raw. Meat and dairy products would be far less harmful consumed raw as they are by some native populations, but most people find the idea of raw meat, chicken, etc, objectionable, and raw dairy products, because of legal germ phobia, unobtainable. But this is as it should be; Nature is trying to tell us something . . .

The pros: Dr Max Garten in his book *The Health Secrets of a Naturopathic Doctor* (1967) described how his health had not much improved by becoming a vegetarian and how this led him to try a completely raw food regime. He said:

"The results were electrifying; within a few days
I felt much stronger with a return of my former

enthusiasm. Many of my patients whom I had been able to convert to this new diet also reported similar results."

Dr Garten observed that putrefactive bacteria in the colon increased not only with the eating of meat but also with the degree of heat used in cooking all food, and with this increase so also did the odiferousness of the stool increase along with the appearance of aches and pains. He said:

"It could only be deduced that certain agents in the diet were either missing or had been altered by the heat. The respective protein content of the vegetarian diet had also been found to be indicative of changes in the intestinal flora, legumes such as beans, lentils, peas etc. equally contributing to the display of putrefactive changes."

Thus, although vegetarians usually are healthier and outlive meat-eaters, they may not maintain very good health or live to a very advanced age if they continually cook their food.

Raw Fruit: the Natural Food of Primates

People become vegetarians to improve their health and extend their lives. Some vegetarians go a step further and consume their food mainly uncooked, while others go even further and limit their diet to fruit, which they claim to be the natural food of man.

Their argument is sound for a number of reasons, but one way or the other it is a fact that, in reasonable variation, fruit can provide the full complement of all required nutrients in adequate quantities, remembering that the requirement for protein and fat are much lower than generally believed. Therefore, instead of being considered merely an accessory to conventional meals, fruit should be considered in its own right as a staple food. The advantages of a fruitarian diet are:

1 It provides complete nourishment with the minimum of extraneous substances capable of 'silting' up the tissues.
2 It is most easily digested, minimizing the energy required for digestion (which is substantial), thereby minimizing total food (kilojoule) requirements.
3 It is palatable.
4 It is easily obtained and easily prepared.
5 It satisfies the appetite when sufficient has been eaten— fruitarians are always lean.
6 Minimum but adequate protein is provided.
7 Minimum but adequate essential fats are provided.
8 Maximum energy is available from what is eaten, with only carbon dioxide and water, which are entirely non-toxic, as the by-products.
9 It provides the body with adequate amounts of pure water.
10 It results in a favorable alkaline internal state.
11 Favorable intestinal flora predominate in the bowel.
12 No constipation occurs.
13 No auto-intoxication occurs.
14 The body detoxifies itself.
15 The blood is clean and low viscosity; there is good circulation with low blood pressure.
16 There is the least wear and tear and the least "silting up" of all the body organs and tissues.

That fruit alone can ideally sustain human health and vigor, even without drinking water, indicates that it indeed provides the basis of man's natural diet. Further substantiation of this view is that there are about forty distinct anatomical, physiological and biological features of humans which show unquestionably that the human body is designed mainly for a fruit diet, notwithstanding the fact that, like all animals, they can survive less successfully on a wide variety of foods. These features range from natural fondness for sweet foods, jaw and teeth structure, salivary secretion, length of digestive tract, size of pancreas, stereo color vision and so on. In fact, in all these respects humans are practically identical today with the other higher primates in the wild which, whenever possible, live on fruit.

Evidence of the suitability of fruit as a staple food and not just as an accessory to the conventional diet is to be seen by observing fruitarians who live entirely on a wide variety of fresh fruit, and who display lean youthful bodies, low blood pressure, clear vision and unimpaired faculties, even with advancing years.

A well-known human peculiarity never before connected with this argument but which provides almost conclusive evidence is that humans, like all primates, are incapable of making vitamin C in their bodies, whereas other animals can (excepting guinea pigs and fruit-eating bats). Basing their argument on this fact, it is strongly advocated by many authorities that people should take large amounts of supplementary Vitamin C to compensate for this "error of Nature", which they put down to an unfavorable mutation in our evolutionary past some millions of years ago. To prove this "unlucky mutation" argument completely wrong, and at the same time prove that man is a natural fruit eater, consider:

1 The only mutations which persist to become a universal feature of a species are favorable ones. Unfavorable mutations cannot possibly do so.

2 A genetic change preventing the synthesis of vitamin C in the body, to become universal to an entire species, must therefore have been, at the time, a favorable change.

3 The only possibility of such a genetic change being favorable is for the species to have been already getting more than adequate vitamin C, and that any more was undesirable.

4 The only source of "excess" vitamin C in Nature is a diet of raw fruit. (Only certain tropical fruits contain such high levels of Vitamin C; many fruits contain only small amounts.)

Therefore it is clear that the human diet ideally should be based mainly on fresh fruit, and that past errors which have led to widespread vitamin C deficiencies are dietary— not genetic—errors.

Obviously some fruits are more nutritious than others, and quality will vary according to the quality of the soil in which they are grown. Commercially grown fruit may contain various levels of insecticide poisons, in which case the fruit should be carefully washed or peeled. At the time of writing, the author had subsisted almost entirely on commercially grown fruit for ten years, all the while working long hours under stress seven days a week, and has maintained excellent health. I have chosen the fruit at random with a preference for tropical fruits, and included dried fruits from time to time without any attempt at being scientific about it. It is probably best not to mix the acid fruits with others eaten at the same time. Some people find they experience digestive upsets when at first they embark on a fruitarian diet. This may be because of mixing incompatible fruits or possibly not chewing them properly. The fruit should be taken as snacks throughout the day, as frequently as desired, rather than conventionally as three substantial meals.

If cooked food is eaten at the same time as fruit, the fruit should be eaten first as it digests quickly and clears out of the way of the other food, which may reside in the stomach for several hours.

It is claimed by some people that a fruitarian diet will eventuate in high blood triglycerides and this is why Nathan Pritikin limited fruit. The increase in triglycerides is supposed to follow elevated levels of blood sugar after eating fruit, but this does not occur when eating whole raw fruit, particularly eaten at whim throughout the day rather than in three large meals. An objection to acid fruits such as citrus and pineapples, particularly if unripe, is that, eaten in excess, the acid may cause erosion in the enamel of the teeth. It is interesting to note here that with good body chemistry and a clean mouth, teeth, like bones, are to a great extent self-repairable. With half my teeth jammed with fillings, maybe they are beyond self-repair, but at my yearly pilot medical checkups I enjoy being told by my doctor I have the arteries and blood pressure of a schoolboy. That makes fruit taste better still, even on a winter's day.

A convert to fruitarianism was the Indian philosopher and statesman Mahatma Gandhi, who after experiencing poor health throughout his youth became a student of nature cure at the age of thirty-two. First he became a vegetarian and then a fruitarian. After six months as a fruitarian, he said (quoted from his book *The Health Guide*):

> "A period of six months is all too short to arrive at any definite conclusions on such a vital matter as a complete change of diet. This, however, I can say, that, during this period, I have been able to keep well where others have been attacked by disease, and my physical as well as mental powers are now greater than before. I may not be able to lift heavy loads, but I can do hard labor for a much longer time without fatigue. I can also do more mental work, and with better persistence and resoluteness. I have tried a fruit diet on many sickly people, invariably with great advantage. My own experience, as well as my study of the subject, has confirmed me in the conviction that a fruit diet is the best one for us."

The Japanese soldier who lived wild in the jungles of the Philippines all those years lived on a natural diet and escaped the degeneration awaiting him back in Japan. In Chapter 3 there is a comparison of the Hunza diet with the Western diet; for a comparison of the jungle diet with the Western diet, refer to the table opposite.

From this comparison it can be seen that notwithstanding the Hunzas physical excellence when compared to ours, they still could have done a lot better!

Dieting for Health

From the foregoing, the subject of dieting for health should require no further explanation; it is obvious that to get results it is necessary to eliminate or drastically curtail from our menus the sort of foods that cause toxemia and lead

	Natural Diet	Western Diet
Kilojoules (calories) for adult male (approx.)	8400 (2000)	14,700 (3500)
Vitamin C (approx.)	3000–9000 mg	100 mg
Other vitamins and minerals	adequate	?
Natural enzymes	ideal	almost nil
Protein % (approx.)	4% (ideal)	15% (hazardous)
Fat % (approx.)	4% (ideal)	40% (dangerous)
Natural carbohydrate % (approx.)	92% (ideal)	5% (inadequate)
Refined carbohydrate % (approx.)	nil	40% (dangerous)
Cholesterol	almost nil	10.4 mmol/l (dangerous)
Fiber	adequate	inadequate
Salt and condiments	nil	hazardous
Caffeine in tea, coffee, soft drinks	nil	hazardous
Preservatives	nil	hazardous
Heat damage to food	nil	hazardous
Chemicals	nil	hazardous

to ill health. This means denying ourselves a certain amount of pleasure in eating, a denial a lot of people refuse to accept on the grounds that they are not overweight and that they have "never had a day's sickness in their life". "Moderation in all things" is another good reason.

Because the Western diet contains adequate quantities of all the nutrients needed to sustain life, it is considered to be "balanced" and capable of maintaining good health. This is true only to a point, because reasonable health can be maintained on the Western diet only as long as the digestive system, liver and other vital organs are capable of enduring the load the diet puts on them in their efforts to provide a pure and complete bloodstream from processed and semi-artificial food.

Dieting for better health then has little to do with taking vitamins, minerals and "health foods", because when it is realized that most of the malnutrition suffered in civilization eventuates not because of diet deficiencies but because it is improperly constituted, then it becomes clear that the first thing to do is to cut out the harmful things. Without making any changes in the diet at all, great improvements in health can be achieved simply by eating less and cutting out salt, so accomplishing a purer bloodstream and at the same time getting rid of excess weight.

Although overweight is associated with increased risk of disease and shortened lifespan, it does not follow that dieting for weight loss and dieting for health are the same. Whereas proper dieting will achieve both weight adjustment and good health together, there are some slimming diets which achieve weight loss at the expense of health. Diets such as the Atkins diet, the Stillman diet and the Scarsdale diet are effective in reducing weight but are dangerous over a period. They work because they cut down (correctly) on fat and refined carbohydrate, but make the mistake of substituting high-protein foods as "filler-uppers", so increasing the intake of protein from a barely tolerable level to an even less tolerable level certain to worsen toxemia and increase the risk of kidney failure and cancer.

Toxemia is the enemy, and lipotoxemia (lipo = fat) is the arch enemy of health. The worst feature of the Western diet is all the fat in it, and therefore regardless of anything else, our main objective must be to drastically reduce the intake of fat. By virtue of unsticking the blood and improving its circulation and oxygen content, great benefits are felt within three or four days. With less impedance to the digestion by fat, putrefaction in the colon is reduced and therefore toxemia from that source is reduced too. As fat severely inhibits the function of the immune system, reduction of fat brings about vastly improved immune function, also within a few days. Regardless of which "health diet" a person chooses, be it the European grape diet, the Pritikin diet, the Gerson diet, the Macrobiotic diet, the fruit juice diet, or just plain fasting, in all cases a great improvement in wellbeing is experienced in three or four days, the improvement being due to the fact that all these diets are low in fat.

Medical authorities, slowly getting the message, currently recommend people should reduce the amount of fat in their diet to thirty per cent but this is nowhere near good enough. Some benefit is felt at twenty per cent but for proper effect the maximum should be ten per cent as has already been described in previous chapters.

There are several alternative methods of reducing fat and cholesterol in the blood. Physical endurance (aerobic) exercise produces what is called the "training effect" by which the body becomes capable of more efficiently metabolizing blood fats for the production of energy. Athletes in training therefore display lower blood viscosity, lower blood pressure, higher oxygen levels, better immune function and better general health when on the conventional Western diet than do untrained people on the same diet. The other way of coping better with high levels of dietary fat (can you guess?) is to eat the fat raw the way the primitive Eskimos do, and allow the adipose lipase (enzyme) in the fat itself to predigest the fat to allow its more thorough breakdown during digestion. Not that the Western diet ever contained much whale blubber, but at least once upon a time the milk, butter and cheese was unpasteurised and contained valuable enzymes. I guess the easiest way to eliminate fat from the bloodstream is simply not to eat it in the first place, remembering that all foods contain some, the bad items being foods of animal origin, dairy products, and of course all extracted vegetable oils and anything containing them. Remember too that the body makes its own fat out of protein and carbohydrates and that when refined carbohydrates, sugar and alcohol are taken, these too will elevate the amount of fat (triglycerides) in the blood. Animal fat of course contains lots of cholesterol too, so eliminating this fat from the diet serves a double purpose.

The next step in dietary improvement of course is to reduce the amount of protein in the diet. Cutting out foods of animal origin—meat, chicken, eggs and dairy products—will achieve this because these foods are the major source of protein in the conventional diet, and by eliminating them you eliminate in one move not only excess protein but cholesterol and excess fat as well. Conventional nutritionalists usually advise vegetarians to maintain their protein intake levels by using nuts, lentils and beans which are high in vegetable protein, but there is absolutely no need for this as our aim is to reduce protein to between five and ten per cent. On the strict vegetarian diet it is difficult to get protein down to five per cent anyhow.

By reducing the worst ingredients of the Western diet—excess fat, excess protein, cholesterol and salt—to safe levels, you will have eliminated to a great extent the factors underlying most of the diseases of modern civilization, particularly atherosclerosis (heart disease), kidney disease and cancer, but it should be pointed out that the substitution of the dangerous fat and cholesterol foods with a lot of grain products can lead to toxemia of a different kind, possibly as harmful as existed beforehand.

Reference back to previous pages will remind you that a lot more improvements can still be made if you are looking for the very best results, because the question comes in two parts: (a) What immediate degree of health do I want? and (b) How long do I want it to last? A moderate dietary change may restore a forty year old to good health, whereas the same change may not get the desired results in a person of sixty whose vital organs are in worse condition. The forty year old, as he gets older, may find he needs to be stricter with his diet to maintain good health. A lot of people claim they don't need to diet for health at all, because they have never had a day's sickness in their life. The trouble is they cannot see the degeneration going on inside them and they don't even feel it until they perhaps one day start getting chest pains or maybe feel a strange lump inside them, or spit out some blood. Thus someone, proud of their vigorous health, may suddenly overnight become a permanent invalid or even be finished for good.

It is human nature to seek pleasure and to put other

things aside until forced to attend to them, and for this reason most people only start thinking of their health when it starts to fail. Then they want a "quick fix" so they can return to their indulgences again. When they find medicine is a waste of time and money they may decide to try diet. There are many diets to choose from. All of them require self-discipline, because to some extent or other the seductive flavors of the Western diet must be abandoned. We are addicted to these flavors and giving them up is as hard as giving up any other drug.

Fad Diets for Health

In Europe, the grape diet has for years been popular in various spas and sanitaria, where sick people go to spend some weeks to recover their failing health. In a short while invalids feel great, lose weight, etc, and then return home to indulge in their favorite foods again, planning on another spa holiday next year.

Other people go on fruit juice fasts, grapefruit diets and so on and get the same wonderful results for just as long as they remain away from the Western-style food. They almost always return to their old eating habits, not because they cannot break the habit but because they cannot break the addiction. Habit and addiction are not the same thing.

In the mid-1800s a wonderful health diet was invented by Dr J. H. Salisbury of New York. It was of course called the Salisbury diet, and so incredibly good were the results gained by it that people travelled even from Europe to be treated by Dr Salisbury. The story of the Salisbury diet is told in a book by Dr Emmet Densmore of England called *How Nature Cures*, written almost one hundred years ago. The writer was astonished to read that the diet consisted of nothing other than lean, partially cooked ground beefsteak taken three times a day preceded an hour beforehand by a pint of hot water and another pint of water taken before retiring at night. On this diet the patients all suffered a constant craving for something sweet, but all rapidly improved in health. Although potentially dangerous in the long term, the diet achieved marvellous short-term results simply because it was low in fat and devoid of starch, starch being from Dr Densmore's experience the worst dietary factor of all. In effect the diet was equivalent to a partial fast, and the European patients could have achieved better results and saved themselves a long trip by going to Germany and eating grapes.

Fasting

For people in well enough condition to undertake a fast this is probably the most rapid and effective way to detoxify the body and return it to full function and health. For best results the fast should continue until the body is completely detoxified and this may take anything from a week or two to several months depending on the individual case. Fasting must be carefully supervised and is outside the scope of this discussion (*see* "Fasting" in Chapter 15).

Health diets for permanent adoption

The Weight Watchers' diet. This diet is calculated more to achieve weight loss than to improve health, but if followed properly both weight loss and improved health will follow. The Weight Watchers' diet could be described as "the Western diet in moderation", and health improvement can be expected mainly as a result of eating fewer kilojoules rather than changing the kind of food. The diet is nowhere near ideal because it still permits too much protein and fat, mayonnaise, cheese, eggs, salt and pepper. But it is better than the conventional Western diet and is a good start in the right direction.

Vegetarian diet. A true vegetarian diet permits no foods of animal origin at all. People following such a diet are known as "vegans". People who eat no animal flesh of any kind (or fish) but include milk, cheese and eggs in their diet are referred to as lacto-ovo vegetarians.

The obvious advantage of vegetarianism is the absence in the diet of animal protein, animal fat and cholesterol. Lacto-ovo vegetarians still take in these harmful substances because dairy products and eggs are high in them, and so they gain only partial benefit.

As a rule, most vegetarians consume a fair amount of cereal (grain) products, lentils and beans and as a result still take in too much protein as well as too much starch. As will be explained later, these foods are of very dubious value although they are widely accepted as "health foods". In addition, further harm ensues when vegetable oils are freely used, and when the vegetarian food is cooked— particularly if overcooked, salted and spiced.

Thus many vegetarians are not much better off, healthwise, than those consuming the traditional diet. However, notwithstanding these mistakes, the advantages of following the vegetarian way of life are still considerable, as demonstrated by statistics of death rates quoted from the medical journal *Circulation*, Vol. 58, No. 1, July 1978. The quotation is from the text of a lecture called "Lifestyles, Major Risk Factors, Proof and Public Policy" by noted cardiologist Dr Jeremiah Stamler.

> "An additional comparison has recently become available, with data on mortality, for three groups of Californian Seventh Day Adventists (non-vegetarian, lacto-ovo-vegetarian and pure vegetarian) compared with the Californian general population. Seventh Day Adventists have lower mean serum cholesterol levels than Americans generally. For 47,000 Seventh Day Adventist men aged 35 and over, age-sex-standardized, mortality rates were 34% lower for non-vegetarians, 57% lower for the lacto-ovo-vegetarians and 77% lower for the pure vegetarians compared to the general population. Seventh Day Adventists differ from the general population in other respects as well, eg abstinence from both alcohol and tobacco.
>
> Since the data from both animal and human studies indicate that high blood pressure and cigarette smoking are minimally significant for atherogenesis in the absence of the nutritional

metabolic prerequisites, it is further reasonable and sound to designate "rich" diet as a PRIMARY, ESSENTIAL, NECESSARY CAUSE of the current epidemic of premature atherosclerotic disease raging in the Western industrialized countries. Cigarette smoking and hypertension are important secondary or complementary causes."

The Macrobiotic diet. Any diet that drastically cuts out fat and cholesterol must, like the Salisbury diet, show good results. The macrobiotic diet, of Japanese origin, endows great health benefits when it is adopted by people who have been on the Western diet. The diet is based on grain products, principally brown rice steam or boiled, which accounts for over fifty per cent of the total intake, about twenty-five per cent cooked vegetables, ten per cent beans or lentils, five per cent miso, five per cent seaweed and only five to ten per cent raw vegetables. Fruit is not recommended and salt is allowed.

The macrobiotic diet is claimed to be a healthy diet and indeed, by comparison to the Western diet, may appear to be so. The diet's shortcomings will be already apparent to the reader and will become even more apparent in later discussion.

The Pritikin diet. Nathan Pritikin claimed his diet to be the "healthiest diet in the world". If he was comparing the Pritikin diet to the traditional diets of the major population groups around the world, his claim would have been substantially correct. There is no question of the Pritikin diet's superiority over the Western diet for a start, and its emphasis on complex carbohydrates and reduction of protein and fat make it theoretically a far better diet than the traditional balanced diet espoused by today's nutritional experts.

The Pritikin diet achieves rapid, often spectacular results, first and foremost because of its very low fat content. It achieves reversal of atherosclerosis because of its low cholesterol content. It achieves reduction of blood pressure by virtue of unsticking the blood and lowering its viscosity, and by the same means permits the body's insulin to work better, so reversing diabetes. Lots of other good things happen simply because of improved circulation and more oxygen in the tissues. But the Pritikin diet too has faults which can lead to trouble if not circumvented, the main fault being that, like the macrobiotic diet, it relies too heavily on grain products and permits too much cooking.

The Gerson diet. Originally devised to solve the problem of migraine, the Gerson diet was found to be effective in arresting other metabolic and degenerative diseases, and has been used with high levels of success in the treatment of cancer since the 1930s. The diet is very low in fat, cholesterol and protein, consisting mainly of raw vegetables, fruit and juices made from these. Some cooked vegetables and rice are permitted, but the diet does not contain much grains and therefore must be considered superior to the Pritikin diet. The results demonstrated by Dr Gerson, and more lately by his daughter Charlotte, clearly demonstrate this superiority.

The Hunza diet. The unsurpassed health and physical endurance of the legendary Hunza race was proven in exhaustive tests by Major General Sir Robert McCarrison, MD, in the 1920s to be directly attributable to the Hunza diet (*The Wheel of Health*, Dr G. T. Wrench; *see also The Health Revolution*). The Hunza diet was similar to the Pritikin diet in that it contained a fair amount of wholegrain foods mainly in the form of wheatmeal bread, hardly any meat or fish, and a lot of vegetables, boiled and raw. As well, however, the diet contained liberal quantities of raw fruit, raw milk and cheese. There were no chickens, eggs, tea, sugar or rice. In the seven years he spent among the Hunzas, Dr McCarrison's medical skills were almost entirely confined to the treatment of accidental lesions, operations for granular eyelids, and the removal of senile cataracts, as other health problems were practically unknown. Dr Wrench, in his account, remarked upon the amount of raw food consumed by the Hunzas and attributed this mainly to be why they were so free of disease.

The raw food diet. Nobody can claim to have invented the raw food diet; it is the diet provided by Mother Nature in the first place. Dr Richard Lambe of England extolled the virtues of the raw vegetarian diet back in 1809, and described the successful use of it in the treatment of cancer patients.

Diets made up of raw fruits and/or raw vegetables have been the key to the success of the famous sanatoria in Europe, USA, Australia and elsewhere for many years. These include the Battle Creek Sanatorium started by Dr Harvey Kellogg of the USA a hundred years ago, the Bircher Benner Sanatorium in Switzerland, the Hopewood Health Centre in Australia and Dr Ann Wigmore's Hippocrates Health Centers in the USA. The advantages of eating food uncooked are many and result in health benefits unobtainable from cooked food. Some foods, such as cereals and potatoes, are difficult to digest uncooked but, as will be explained later, such foods are of dubious value anyway and are better left alone.

The fruitarian diet. Theoretically, and in practice, a diet composed of high quality, ripe, raw fruits provides the human body with all the nutrients it needs with the very least expenditure of digestive effort, at the same time producing no toxic by-products and so allowing the body to detoxify itself and perform at its peak. Raw fruits are more palatable and provide more energy for a given amount than vegetables and can be prepared with less effort and less waste. Not only can the highest level of health be attained on a fruitarian diet but, because it places so much less wear and tear on the body's vital organs, degeneration is slowed down and the lifespan extended.

The facts and fallacies of "health foods"
When you walk into a health food store and look around, what do you see? One wall of shelves is packed with vitamins

and mineral products, all expensive and all unnecessary for people on a reasonable diet. Another section displays jars of seaweed extracts, sea salt, vegetable salts, lecithin granules and so on, all of which have dubious value. Seaweed undoubtedly contains minerals that may be light on in some people's diet, but sea salt, apart from the fact it contains iodine, an essential trace mineral missing from the soil in a few areas of the world, is still plain sodium chloride, which is common salt—a dangerous product. Vegetable salt is a flavoring powder made from vegetable extracts but has little flavor of its own and so when you read the label on the jar it usually reveals the fact that ordinary salt or sea salt forms part of the mixture.

Then you see nuts of all kinds, dried lentils, soya beans—bins full of them—foods which contain high levels of fat and protein and are stressful to the digestive system. Shelves are stacked with bottles of polyunsaturated vegetable oils—100 per cent fat—which although containing no cholesterol as do animal fats, nevertheless cause red cell and platelet aggregation in the blood and are associated with increased risk of cancer.

Cookies, biscuits and energy bars, some of which are high in fat and sugar and none of which are as healthful as a good banana. Bins of brown rice and other grains— fair enough foods if eaten sparingly—and bins of dried fruits. Dried fruits, if they are sun dried and unsulphered, are good foods but they are very concentrated and better eaten sparingly as snacks when fresh fruit is not available.

One food item which could be considered as a health-promoting food is garlic, not because it provides valuable nutrients the body needs, but because of its therapeutic medicinal property in a body handicapped by a high-fat diet. Garlic, onions and other herbal extracts such as vitamin E have the effect of unsticking the blood to permit improved circulation. Used for this purpose these products are more medicines than foods, but at least garlic tastes good.

The contents of health food stores can be considered health giving only to the extent they are less harmful than meat, chicken and dairy products. The only foods that qualify to be called health foods, using the true meaning of the word 'health', are fresh fruits and vegetables; you can maintain good health indefinitely on these but the same cannot be said for the general run of foods available in health food stores.

Summarizing health diets

Apart from observing the fact that in general the cooking of food leads to an overworked digestive system and increased toxemia, the single common denominator possessed by all effective health diets, cooked or raw, is the drastic lowering of the fat content, which allows the bloodstream to clear itself of fat and allows the red blood cells and blood platelets to unstick, so reducing the blood viscosity and permitting its free circulation and oxygen-carrying ability. The enormous improvement in wellbeing that results from this single factor of improved blood condition has nothing to do with anything contained in the diet—the benefit stems from what has been taken out of the diet.

So great is the improvement of health and wellbeing achieved by the simple expedient of improving the circulation that the beneficiaries think they have struck the jackpot; they think they have discovered the perfect diet, be it the grape diet, the macrobiotic diet, the Pritikin diet, the Gerson diet or maybe even the Salisbury diet. And this is easy to understand, but there is more to good health than just improving the blood circulation. What about the delicate chemistry of the blood? What about the avoidance of toxemia? The wear and tear on our internal organs? The wastage of digestive energy and valuable enzymes?

Insidious degeneration can continue undetected in a body apparently brimming with vigorous health. Probably the best example of this is the constant occurrence of sudden death by heart attack of extremely fit athletes and runners. Right up until their sudden collapse, which usually occurs during or just after vigorous activity, these people display all the signs of good health. Their blood viscosity is low because they can metabolize fat quickly from their blood and so their blood pressure is good, they feel good because their blood contains plenty of oxygen, and they don't "catch" colds because their immune systems are performing properly. They are healthy in this sense, but when death overtakes them autopsies reveal coronary arteries blocked with cholesterol. They had been under the illusion that endurance exercise prevents heart disease, but the evidence is now clear that physical training does not prevent the accumulation of dietary cholesterol in the arteries; it merely maintains a better blood flow and prevents the usual symptoms of heart disease from being displayed.

Nathan Pritikin was the first one to loudly warn the public of the dangerous illusion that athletes could indulge in a high-cholesterol diet and get away with it. But there are other illusions of which Pritikin was not aware. Avoiding heart disease is not the be all and end all in the quest for good health.

Clean arteries and thin blood are the prime essentials and these are easily accomplished on the Pritikin diet providing the diet is properly followed. The next step is attending to the actual chemistry of the blood and how perfect chemistry can be achieved with the least wear and tear on the vital organs. This involves further investigation into nutrition and the enzymes that make improved nutrition possible. The subject becomes a little different from that of dieting for immediate health benefits, it becomes one of gaining long-term benefit—that is—*dieting for longevity*.

Dieting for Longevity

Do tissues and organs wear out, or are they gradually destroyed by processes which could possibly be avoided? Scientific opinion agrees that the human life span potential is about 120 years, and some estimates go higher. These estimates are probably conservative, because quite a number of people are known to have exceeded 110 years without making any special efforts at all to preserve themselves. Be that as it may, the consensus of opinion is that by taking reasonable care, the degeneration which constitutes the aging process can be slowed down so that old age is postponed.

Old age defined

Old age is a degenerative disease of the entire body, the progress of which is determined more by the degenerating factors in a person's lifestyle than by their chronological age.

Old age described

Everyone knows what old age looks like from the outside, but what changes occur inside the body? In his book *The Span of Life*, Dr William Malisoff described the atrophy and degeneration of every organ and tissue in the body that accompanies old age and the malfunctions which occur as a result. He said:

> "The system of organs is so thoroughly connected that all these changes have mutual repercussions. Thus too the liver, pancreas, spleen, kidneys, urinary organs, become atrophied, hardened and degenerated. The capsule of the kidney is thickened, the parenchyma hardened; the connective tissue scleroses and compresses tubules and glomeruli, impairing their action. The changes in the brain, in the spinal cord, in the nerves, are of a similar character.
>
> The description of the changes would fill many volumes. We can summarize that they fall into several classes: the atrophies, which have been commented on; the fibroses as replacements by fiber; pigmentations; metaplasias; hyperkeratoses, or skin changes and the like; renunciation of functions, as those of the germ cells and the instance of fat cells which no longer store fat."

Dr Arnold Lorand of Austria, in his book *Old Age Deferred*, described old age as a condition in which there is a diminution of metabolism, ie the assimilation and conversion of food into energy, and is characterized by the abundant growth of connective tissue in vital organs, diminution of oxidation and increased auto-intoxication.

Dr Charles de Lacy Evans of England in his book *How to Prolong Life: an Enquiry into the Cause of Old Age and Natural Death*, written one hundred years ago, was more specific; he said:

> "The most marked feature in old age is that fibrinous, gelatinous and earthy deposit has taken place in the system; the latter being chiefly of phosphate and carbonate of lime, with small quantities of sulphate of lime, magnesia and traces of other earths."

He added that the deposits occur in all tissues, including the bones and blood vessels, which harden and reduce in caliber, and quoted a Doctor C. J. B. Williams, who said:

> " 'The process is, therefore, to be viewed as almost entirely of a chemical nature, and as consisting of the concretion and accumulation of calcareous salts, phosphate and carbonate of lime in the debris of animal matter.' "

Dr de Lacy Evans went on to explain how the fibrinous, gelatinous substances were formed by the oxidation within the bloodstream and tissues of excessive albumin (protein), and how the earthy deposits were derived mainly from grain products and root and leafy vegetables and to a lesser extent from animal products. Dr Evans tended to blame the formation of the fibrinous, gelatinous substances on the presence of oxygen, just as some biochemists do today with their 'free radical' theory of aging. More pertinent to the argument, in the author's opinion, is that if the diet is correct then neither the excess albumin nor the free radicals will present themselves in the first place to improperly use the body's valuable oxygen.

Dr Arthur C. Giese, Professor of Biology Emeritus, Stanford University, in his book *Living with Our Sun's Ultraviolet Rays* said:

> "In our multi-cellular bodies some cells, such as those of the epidermal basal layer, continue to divide

throughout life; others—for example nerve and
muscle cells—differentiate and cease dividing at
birth. Nevertheless, they continue to function for
a lifetime, with gradually lessening activity and
progressively filling with insoluble wastes and
pigments."

As the tissues slowly acquire these characteristics of
old age their decline is further characterized by, and is
measurable by, a corresponding decrease in enzyme levels
and activity. On the other hand, animal tissue cells grown
in cultures in the laboratory, properly cleansed and drained,
do not degenerate in this fashion and may outlast the animal
from which they originated many times over. It is held
by some researchers (at least in theory) that in ideal
circumstances immortality is possible. Other experiments
with live animals fed on minimum rations showed
improved health and a life extension of fifty to one hundred
per cent over that of unrestricted control animals on the
same diet.

The longest lived populations in the world are
accepted generally to be the people of Hunza in northern
Pakistan, Vilcabamba in Ecuador, and Georgia in Russia.
An analysis of these peoples' living habits carried out under
the auspices of the *National Geographic* in 1971 by Dr
Alexander Leaf of New York provided a good reason why
they outlived people of the Western world. The traditional
diets of these long-lived (by our standards) people contained
only half to two thirds the kilojoules of the average
American intake, about a quarter the amount of fat and
half the protein. Their carbohydrate intake was about the
same but was unprocessed instead of processed. As well,
these people got more outdoor exercise and were less subject
to stress than Americans.

In his book, Dr de Lacy Evans when reviewing a study
of centenarians in England in the 19th Century said:

"On reviewing nearly 2,000 reported cases of persons
who lived more than a century, we generally find
some peculiarity of diet or habits to account for
their alleged longevity; we find some were living

amongst all the luxuries life could afford, others in the most abject poverty—begging their bread; some were samples of symmetry and physique, others cripples; some drank large quantities of water, others little; some were total abstainers from alcoholic drinks, other drunkards; some smoked tobacco, others did not; some lived entirely on vegetables, others to a great extent on animal foods; some led active lives, others sedentary; some worked with their brain, others with their hands; some ate only one meal a day, others four or five; some few ate large quantities of food, others a small amount; in fact, we notice great divergence both in habits and diet, but in those cases where we have been able to obtain a reliable account of the diet, we find one *great cause* which accounts for the majority of cases of longevity, *moderation in the quantity of food.*"

Thus perhaps the first rule in dieting for longevity is to eat sparingly, whatever the make up of the diet. Even on a bad diet this rule will still permit better health and extended life because less wear and tear will have to be endured by the body.

So it becomes clear that "old age" occurs because we take into our bodies, mainly via food, harmful substances which overtax the digestive system, cause toxemia of the *milieu interieur*, overtax the eliminatory organs, and to a greater or lesser extent gradually accumulate in the tissues and cells to increasingly impede their functions.

It follows then that old age can be deferred by selecting foods which provide the best nutrition with the least digestive effort and the least amount of harmful residues, and consuming such foods in great moderation.

In Conclusion on Longevity

That "a man is an old as his arteries" was stated first by the 17th-Century physician Thomas Sydenham. That "a man's arteries are as old as he makes them" was stated by Robert Bell, a 19th-Century physician. Perhaps we can proceed one step further to state the obvious: "The arteries and all the organs and tissues are as young as the cells of which they are made and the milieu interieur which sustains them."

Diet is not the only factor in longevity, of course, but it is by far the main one. The closer we can get to an ideal diet and maintain it, the less will be the wear and tear on our organs and the slower the accumulation of the fibrinous, gelatinous growths and calcareous mineral salts in our cells and tissues.

Think of all those little cells. Says Dr Edward J. Stiegbitz, MS MD FACP, in his book *The Second Forty Years:*

> "Superficially, the answer is simple; intrinsically, extremely complex. Whether the cells themselves are, or are not, potentially immortal is largely beside the point. The essential fact is that continuance of such perpetual youth, as displayed by Carrel's chick heart cultures[1], is absolutely dependent upon the maintenance of *an ideal environment.* Cultures must be aseptically transplanted to fresh media at frequent intervals or growth stops and the cells die, poisoned by the accumulating chemical debris of their living, and starved because their foodstuffs are used up. Contamination with even minute amounts of toxic substances or any inadequacy of any one of many nutritional requisites immediately interrupts the marvellous lifestream. **The quality of the cellular environment is the determining factor,** *whether the cells be growing in vitro in a test-tube, or in vivo, in the living and functioning organism.*"

[1] In 1912 Dr Alexis Carrel of the Rockefeller Institute, New York, kept alive some cells taken from the heart tissue of an embryo chicken. Properly nourished and cleansed, the cell culture thrived and appeared to be immortal, at least until 1947 when the experiment was terminated.

Your body is a living and functioning organism and you want it to stay that way. We know what to do. We have discussed at great length the factors responsible for polluting the *milieu interieur* of the body, and to eliminate them would appear to be easier said than done. Not everybody can arrange to live in a tropical Garden of Eden.

We can only do our best with what we have available, and the first step, wherever your live, is to cut down on the things that do the most harm. Eat as much as you can of your food raw. Cut out salt. Think of those little cells. Think of how clean your arteries will be, how comforting it will be never to worry about cancer. Each step you take will improve your wellbeing and increase your life expectancy.

Think of fruit as sustaining food and not just as an accessory adding color to the sideboard, although it is admitted that much of the commercially grown fruit available today looks a lot better than it tastes. Lack of taste means lack of nutrition and possibly at the same time the presence of insecticide traces. Quality is important.

Do the best you can, remembering Dr de Lacy Evans' words of wisdom:

> "There is, therefore, a simplicity, a reason, a wonderful philosophy in the first command given to man—Man may live entirely upon fruits in better health than the majority of mankind now enjoy. Good, sound, ripe fruits are never the cause of disease, but the vegetable acids, as we have before stated, lower the temperature of the body, decrease the process of combustion or oxidation—therefore the waste of the system—less sleep is required, activity is increased, fatigue or thirst is hardly experienced; still the body is well nourished, and as a comparatively small quantity of earth salts are taken into the system, the cause of old age is in some degree removed, the effect is delayed, and life is prolonged to a period far beyond our 'threescore and ten'."

"There is little question any more that artery plaque reversal can for the first time be considered possible." Dr Nash in *Circulation*, official journal of the American Heart Association, September 1977.

"With a cholesterol level of 150 [3.9] or less, plaque reversal in two years is possible." Dr R. Wissler, Chicago Medical School, addressing the American Heart Association, June 1977.

"The three major killers in modern society, Coronary Heart Disease, Cancer and Strokes, can all be linked to what people eat and drink." Dr B. Hetzel, Chief of the CSIRO Division of Human Nutrition and Foundation Professor of Social and Preventive Medicine, Monash University.

"The major cancers of our time are diet-caused, mainly by fat and cholesterol." Dr Ernst Wynder, American Health Foundation, addressing the USA Government Senate Select Committee on Nutrition and Human Needs.

"With this kind of approach diet only, 80% of diabetics in this country could be normal in 30 to 90 days." Dr James Anderson, University of Kentucky Medical Centre.

"Progressive pernicious anaemia, asthma, Bright's disease, diabetes, rheumatism, arthritis, neuritis, gastric or duodenal ulcer, every form of digestive disturbance, eczema, psoriasis, pityriasis, goitres of all types, tumors, tuberculosis—any and all of these varied forms of so-called disease fall under one head, chemical imbalance of the body, and all subject to restoration to the normal through correction of the body chemistry and thorough drainage." William Howard Hay, MD (from *The New Health Era*, 1933).

CHAPTER 15

Reversing the Diseases of Civilization

We are not concerned with diseases but with mistakes . . . of living. Get rid of the mistakes and the diseases will disappear of their own accord.

Dr Are Waerland

The mistakes of living built into our civilized way of life that together lead to the metabolic malfunctions we call disease have already been described in previous chapters, but as some misconceptions or doubts may still exist a little more information will not go astray, if only to counteract some of the erroneous views expounded by the various experts, for instance, that grain products are wonder foods or that wonder drugs are a boon to mankind. Misguidance abounds.

Because of misguidance by "experts" on nutrition, a great many health-conscious people get arthritis or even cancer (which is the reason *Improving on Pritikin* was written), and because of further misguidance by medical experts a lot of these health-conscious people perish. The misguidance stems from the entrenched concept of the "five major food groups" which concept, even modified to reduce fat levels from forty per cent to thirty per cent of total food kilojoules, still guarantees lipotoxemia by way of excess fat and protein. Whereas nutritional misguidance results from the misinterpretation of information that is reasonably accurate, medical misguidance is far worse because not only does it stem from established beliefs that are entirely erroneous, not only are the so-called experts ignorant and confused about what they are supposedly expert in, not only therefore is the guidance they offer hopelessly in error, but the guidance is all the more dangerous because dressed in the dignified terms that doctors use to "impress the natives", it is accepted with complete trust by the unsuspecting patient.

Remember Dr Mendelsohn's advice from Chapter 10. "There's no more dangerous activity than walking into a doctor's office, clinic, or hospital unprepared . . ."

Steering clear of doctors when your body is not working properly does not mean you must undertake self-treatment for disease, however, because as Dr Waerland proclaimed: "We are not concerned with diseases . . . but with mistakes of living. Get rid of the mistakes and the diseases will disappear of their own accord." In other words: correct the mistakes, purify the *milieu interieur*, restore homeostasis, and there you have it—glowing health again. No tests, no drugs, no trauma, no expense.

The many factors causing toxemia and the loss of homeostasis are listed in previous chapters, and it is according to the sort of dietary errors and to a lesser extent the other errors and their degree that the corresponding symptoms of impaired homeostasis are displayed. It is conventional of course to regard a symptom as a specific disease in its own right and to give it a name, and as there are innumerable variations in the way homeostasis can be impaired, so in the medical textbooks appear innumerable names of diseases, it being considered the peak of medical skill to diagnose correctly which is which, even though a doctor has no idea of the cause and no idea of how to "cure" whatever it is called. But as can be seen, that while each different symptom or group of symptoms can point to the errors underlying them, the procedure of diagnosis is completely superfluous because in all cases all that needs to be done is to restore homeostasis, and once health returns who cares what name belonged to the now vanished "disease"?

It must be remembered that the Western diet conveys toxemia in a double-barrelled form called lipotoxemia due to the high levels of fat that enters the bloodstream, so that the *milieu interieur* is confounded not only chemically, but physically as well. Therefore it should be borne in mind that while homeostasis and good health may in many cases be regained simply by correcting the physical component of toxemia (ie the blood fats that make the blood sticky), for the newfound health to be complete and lasting the chemical component needs to be corrected as well. Regarding the chemical component, it should be remembered that apart from the toxemia produced from by-products of excess protein, fat, etc in the diet, toxins from other sources may contribute heavily, for instance: mercury from amalgam tooth fillings, infected teeth, fluoride, chlorine, etc in drinking water, residual hormones used in beef production, residual chemicals in food crops, air pollution and so on.

It must also be remembered that all chemical functions in the body, both for normal metabolism and for detoxification, are entirely dependent on enzymes. The more work to be done, the more enzymes are required. To make enzymes, the body needs colloidal minerals of all kinds, the best source of which, by far, are fresh, raw fruit and vegetables.

Apparent Causes and Apparent Cures

The body has an enormous capacity, even in old age, to maintain homeostasis in the presence of many harmful influences, and so a reasonable state of "marginal" health can exist which is a borderline condition maybe displaying signs of impending trouble but not yet displaying recognizable symptoms. In the absence of symptoms it is usually assumed that a person is in good health when they are nowhere near it, their borderline condition making them susceptible to infection, allergy or some metabolic upset, from the first adverse influence encountered, and when sickness "attacks" it will be that particular influence (the straw that broke the camel's back) that will get all the blame. Often a person with latent cancer will develop cancer at the site of an injury or bruise, and it is often thought that injury can cause cancer. Likewise cancer may develop following severe emotional stress, or similar stress can bring on an attack of asthma, rheumatoid arthritis, diabetes or angina, but for these "diseases" to occur the body first must be in a highly toxic, borderline condition. It takes a lot of straws to break a camel's back and all must take their share of the blame.

Thus, when someone with multiple sclerosis, cancer, arthritis or similar goes "into remission" for a while only to later suffer another progression of the disease, and then with a bit of luck experience another period of "remission", it is because the balance of factors underlying the degree of toxemia in the body is teetering first one side and then the other of the borderline of the body's capacity to maintain homeostasis. Sometimes something as simple as a little TLC (tender loving care) or confidence inspired by a caring doctor or a faith healer, or simple loss of appetite for food, will swing the balance the right way. When people take garlic, aloe vera, ginseng or something else that lowers blood viscosity (leeches and snake venom extracts can do the same), beneficial effects are experienced if the right side of borderline is regained, whereupon the "curative" effects of these things become part of folklore and "alternative medicine", while they are called quackery by the medical profession because they are not "scientific". Food allergy is another problem which is not consistent and is more severe if a person is fatigued or highly stressed, so before spending weeks testing for "guilty" foods, the main effort should be devoted to fully restoring the body's capacity to maintain homeostasis and adequate production of digestive enzymes.

Alternative Medicine

Under the heading of alternative medicine comes orthomolecular medicine, acupuncture, osteopathy, homeopathic medicine, faith healing, transcendental meditation, chiropractic and so on. All of these practices are forms of "medicine" aimed therapeutically to cure some sort of health problem, and indeed they are all recorded as having achieved either relief from various conditions of disease or in some cases complete "cures", which explains why each method is claimed by its enthusiasts to be the way to go.

But none of these methods achieve permanent "cures", simply because they address only part of a patient's problem without getting to the root of it—toxemia. But even if they don't get very good or lasting results, at least they are a form of medicine that does no harm and doesn't cost a small fortune at every attendance.

Sitting crosslegged in pyramid structures, watching pendulums, or performing Oriental exercises in the open air may make a lot of people feel good but will do little to correct the toxemia within them which is due to the sort of food they eat. An interesting event happened about ten years ago, not long after the author's first book, *The Health Revolution*, was published. A friend of mine, an ex-Air Force pilot, had a flourishing business conducting the practice of pain relief using laserbeam acupuncture. He had a steady clientele because his pain relief treatment worked and his patients kept coming back. When my friend became enthused by the contents of *The Health Revolution* he began to purchase the books by the carton, insisting to his patients they should follow the advice contained therein. To make a short story even shorter, most of his patients changed their diets, lost their pains, and my friend closed up shop and went back to flying airplanes.

What We Want

We are not interested in medicine of any kind—"allopathic" or "alternative". We are not interested in their mediocre achievements in partially restoring health, where patients remain forever borderline with bottles of pills always within easy reach.

We want homeostasis, 100 per cent, with the glowing health that accompanies it, regardless of stress or cold or wind or rain. To avoid the diseases of civilization is simple: you just discard from your lifestyle the factors that cause them, and we already know what they are. To reverse the diseases of civilization is just as simple, and the procedure is exactly the same but with lesser leeway for occasional relaxing of the rules.

Fasting

The quickest and most effective way to detoxify the body and restore complete homeostasis is to go on a fast, where for an indefinite time only pure water is consumed, the length of the fast being dependent on the degree to which the body is encumbered throughout its tissues with accumulated waste products it had been unable in the past to eliminate. In a few days much relief of symptoms is experienced because blood fats quickly diminish and circulation greatly improves, but this is only the beginning, and in some cases fasts have been extended for many weeks before complete detoxification is achieved. While the fast is in progress no hunger pangs are suffered and the body's metabolism is sustained on body fat and superfluous tissue, as the organs of elimination proceed to "clean house". Fasting is not starvation and although the patient may lose a lot of weight and become quite thin, no damage is caused and all systems continue to improve. The signal to end the fast is when the coating disappears from the tongue and unpleasant body odors cease while at the same time a keen appetite returns. By this time the body will have shed whatever symptoms were troubling it such as arthritis, asthma, migraine, angina, diabetes and so on because these problems do not exist in the presence of complete homeostasis.

There are cases of course where a patient may be so depleted in reserves that a fast may be inadvisable, in which case partial fasting, taking only juices of fruits and vegetables (separately) will achieve the desired result.

It is suggested that if a fast is contemplated the subject of fasting should be studied beforehand and the fast should be conducted under supervision in a proper sanatorium. This of course involves time and expense, so unless the situation requires such drastic measures the detoxification program can be simply incorporated into a normal lifestyle with strict attention to natural diet.

There is no specific diet for the correction of any particular health problem you may have, because all health upsets, whatever their nature, stem from unbalanced body chemistry, and so the only object of the exercise is to correct the dietary errors that have led to this imbalance.

The guidelines for correct eating are given in the chapters on Toxemia and Dieting for Health, and providing these guidelines are followed your diet need not be spelled out in a series of ritualistic menus, but can be as varied and interesting as you wish. To assist in preparing simple food to make it more appealing to the eye and palate, there are a number of recipe books available, such as Toni Bobbin's *Anti-Cancer, Anti-Heart Attack, Cookbook*, which make the transition from traditional foods to toxemia-free foods easy.

When toxemia is eliminated and homeostasis restored within the body there is no metabolic malfunction (disease) that will not be corrected by the body's own capacity to heal itself, providing of course that this capacity has not already been irreparably damaged, and this is very rarely the case. There is only one catch to this panacea of free and lasting health, and that is it takes a certain amount of willpower to take advantage of it, because the addiction to the tantalising flavors of our traditional foods is very difficult to abandon, salt being probably the worst of them. But to repeat—there is no health problem that cannot be relieved and, in most cases, completely eliminated by getting rid of the mistakes of living.

The Mental Factor

Just as mental acuity is affected one way or the other by the condition of the blood and general fitness of the body, so too does the reverse apply—the physical status of health can be enormously influenced, for good or for bad, by mental attitude.

It is now fairly well understood how mental stress causes the release of hormones and fatty acids, etc into the bloodstream to cope with a potential "fight or flight" situation, but more complex is the interaction of mind and body involving the will to live, which although normally programmed for survival can in some circumstances be reversed, and either way can vary greatly in intensity. On one hand you have the case of someone beyond all hope of survival simply refusing to die, and fighting their way up again, and on the other hand you have someone in reasonable physical health but, miserable and with nothing to live for, who just sickens and dies. A better example of how negative thoughts can kill is the way Aboriginals who have broken tribal laws can be punished by the ritual of bone pointing, after which ritual the victim simply wastes away and dies.

The placebo effect of dummy medicines, well known in medical research circles, is put to good use by some doctors loath to inflict drugs upon their patients and who have discovered their patients do just as well taking dummy pills as they do taking real ones. The patients don't know the pills are dummies and the knowledgeable doctor knows in most cases that they will recover with or without medicine anyway, but that their belief in the "cure" will help them do so more quickly.

As mentioned earlier, the belief system can work both

ways. It is the doctor's job to instil the belief in the patient because without the belief there can be no result, and if for some reason the patient believes that the "medicine" will produce a harmful result, then any effect produced will indeed be harmful. For instance if a patient takes a placebo in the belief it is a drug that produced a skin rash to them in the past, or perhaps nausea, then the chemically inert placebo is capable of reproducing these same symptoms.

At the World Health conference on Asian medicine in Canberra in 1979, a Tibetan woman doctor, Dr Losang Dolma, described how she achieved an eighty per cent success rate in treating cancer using precious stones ground up and made into pills. The director of the New South Wales Cancer Council was reluctant to comment at the time, saying it was a far-fetched notion but he was willing to learn. It is to be hoped that he did learn something, because if someone is to recover from any illness, especially cancer, their mental attitude is of paramount importance.

The entire history of medicine is a mixture of confusion and argument about what is scientific and what is quackery. Had Losang Dolma come from a Sydney suburb instead of Tibet, she would have long before been jailed as a cancer quack.

The many claims made over the years that various mixtures of herbs, roots, etc were effective cancer cures cannot be swept aside as unscientific because many of them achieved their purpose, according to the personal testimonies produced to support them. Homeopathy is a branch of alternative medicine based on potions containing ingredients in quantities so miniscule (sometimes in the order of a trillionth of a grain) that it seems absolutely impossible for the medicine to produce the slightest effect even on an insect. But homeopathy has many supporters, even from the ranks of medical doctors, the reason being that they have seen results beneficial to the patients so treated. Notwithstanding that herbs and so on could perhaps provide the patient's body with some nutrient it may have been lacking, it is as likely as not that the benefits when sometimes gained have been via mental pathways.

Some patients respond to treatments better than others, and it was Sir William Osler (1849-1919), the great British physician, who is quoted as saying: "It is more important to know what kind of patient has the disease than to know what kind of disease the patient has."

And well Sir William could have added: "It is more important what kind of doctor a patient has than what kind of medicine the doctor employs."

In his book *Getting Well Again* (1978), Dr Carl Simonton described dramatic remissions of cancer in patients he had taught to visualise the white cells of their immune systems as an army attacking their cancer cells and destroying them. Dr Simonton said: "You are more in charge of your life—and even the development and progress of a disease, such as cancer—than you may realize. You may actually, through a power within you, be able to decide whether you live or die."

Dr Harry A. Hoxsey, a cancer specialist from Dallas, Texas in the 1930s and 40s, said in his book *You Don't Have To Die*: "Tell a victim he is hopeless (or let him discover it from his family) and the will to live becomes paralyzed. Show him a way out, strip him of fear and hysteria, give him even a forlorn hope, and the will to live is stimulated. It becomes a powerful ally in the battle against death."

The favorable influence of faith and positive thinking in influencing the body's metabolism to function better is called "faith healing", and if as a result of it homeostasis is restored sufficiently for the symptoms of disease to regress, it is sometimes claimed that a miracle cure has been performed when all that has happened is a natural physiological response to a favorable mental influence. The patient has not been "cured" at all, but merely assisted back to the right side of a borderline condition, hopefully to remain there. Of course, for the healing process to be fully accomplished the *milieu interieur* must be purified as well.

Norman Cousins, a veteran journalist and author,

created a great deal of awareness in the medical profession about the power of the mind affecting the course of a disease with his book *Anatomy of an Illness* (Bantam, 1979), in which he described how he overcame a so-called "terminal" disease called "ankylosing spondylitis" by removing himself from hospital, declining medical treatment, and instead spending his time watching old comedy movies, meditating, resting, and taking megadoses of vitamin C. He was on his feet again in eight days and he was able soon afterwards to resume work and play tennis and golf again. That all happened in 1964, and so impressed were some of Cousin's influential doctor friends that he ended up lecturing on the mental aspect of medicine at the University of California, Los Angeles.

In December 1980, Cousins, then aged sixty-five, had an almost fatal heart attack and, declining medical advice for bypass surgery, he once again decided to make a recovery by natural healing assisted by his powerful positive mental approach, exercise and modified diet. In this he succeeded, as he described in his next book *The Healing Heart* (1983). However, his triumph lasted only for ten years; his second heart attack was a fatal one.

Notwithstanding that misfortune, Cousins' claims about the immense value of positive, confident optimism in recovery from illness are absolutely correct, and his books are an inspiration to anybody, sick or well.

In *Anatomy of an Illness* Cousins tells of a meeting he had in Africa with Dr Albert Schweitzer, musician, physician and Nobel Prize winner. Replying to Cousins' question as to how the African tribal witchdoctors got such good results, Dr Schweitzer replied: "It's supposed to be a professional secret, but I'll tell you anyway. The witchdoctor succeeds for the same reason all the rest of us succeed. Each patient carries his own doctor inside him. They come to us not knowing the truth. We are at our best when we give the doctor who resides within each patient a chance to go to work." (Lesson 1 for all medical students.)

Cousins used this reference to the "doctor within" to illustrate his chapter devoted to the placebo effect—the power of the mind—and it was a good illustration, but it is doubtful that Dr Schweitzer intended people should think the power of the mind was the only consideration. Years before Schweitzer had made a complete recovery from diabetes, and his wife had made a complete recovery from tuberculosis, but this had only been possible when they had implemented the dietary advice given them by their friend, Dr Max Gerson (*see* Chapter 12 and "Improving on Pritikin" in Chapter 8). They had detoxified their bodies.

Norman Cousins did a good job beating the conventional medical odds, but he could have done better. If in addition to his mental self-conditioning he had adopted the Gerson diet, he could have completely reversed his coronary disease and still be alive today, perhaps to compare notes on physical fitness with Rolet de Castella (Chapter 15).

The Role of Physical Exercise

That regular physical exercise conveys protection against disease is indicated by the fact that it makes people feel better, sleep better and tend to eat less, and by the fact that physically active people tend to live longer than the average. Not only that, but the records show that fit athletes in general suffer less from respiratory infections, breathing problems, diabetes, arthritis, multiple sclerosis, heart attacks, etc, and that the incidence of cancer among them is only one seventh of the average incidence.

These comparisons of athletes with non-athletes are applicable to people in the Western countries, where typically both athletes and non-athletes all consume the traditional foods of the Western diet, so it is clear that the health protection provided by adequate physical exercise is gained by its effect of reducing lipotoxemia, the main underlying cause of all the diseases of the Western world.

The protective effect of sustained and reasonably vigorous exercise by people on the Western diet is multifold:

1 The "training effect" of aerobic exercise relates to the changes that take place within the cells of exercised muscles which enable the muscles to more efficiently use blood fats as a fuel source and to more efficiently utilize the oxygen available to them.

2 With less fat in the blood, the blood is less sticky and therefore lower in viscosity, enabling it to flow better, particularly in partially blocked blood vessels, thus reducing the pumping effort required by the heart.

3 The more vigorous circulation of blood that occurs with exercise helps to keep the arteries supple and expanded, while at locations where artery blockage due to fat and cholesterol have occurred, the demands for increased circulation while exercising cause the increased development of collateral blood vessels around the blockage.

4 Not only is the vigor of blood circulation increased by exercise, but so too is the vigor of the lymph circulation so that toxemia due to a stagnant lymph is cleared and at the same time cells are better nourished.

Thus the resultant improved condition of the blood and lymph fluid greatly enhance an improperly fed body's efforts to maintain homeostasis, with the consequent diminished likelihood of the diseases to which it would be otherwise susceptible.

However, exercise, while enhancing general circulation, does not prevent the build-up of atherosclerosis within the arteries and so a point is reached where exercise eventually becomes dangerous. Usually warning of this danger in the form of angina (chest pains) and breathlessness upon exertion occurs, but sometimes in an extremely fit person there is no early warning at all and a massive heart attack out of the blue is the only symptom they get. As previously explained, extremely fit athletes with blocked coronary arteries have such a development of small but numerous collateral vessels, that while blood viscosity is reasonable their heart muscles are still plentifully supplied with blood, but when the blood's viscosity for some reason becomes so high it cannot pass through the fine collaterals at all, suddenly the heart muscle is so deprived of blood that is stops.

The reason that this catastrophic event so often occurs after a period of strenuous exercise and not during the exercise is because the effect of sustained vigorous exercise is to greatly increase the number of platelets (clotting particles) in the blood, and this is a perfectly natural physiological event, but on top of blood viscosity already elevated by perhaps last night's wine and civilized dinner, the viscosity reaches disaster level. In this way many a confident sportsman has discovered physical fitness is no guarantee of long life.

Thus the role of physical exercise in protecting against the diseases of civilization is a real but limited one which works only to partially correct harmful factors which should not be there in the first place.

But even in the complete absence of the beforementioned harmful factors and in a state of perfect health, regular exercise, even light exercise, is highly desirable in order to ensure good lymph circulation not only to the muscles but throughout the entire body. The *milieu interieur* cannot remain pure if it becomes stagnant, so if someone is incapacitated and immobile it is important they be encouraged to move as much as possible, or massaged, to keep the lymph moving.

How Much Exercise is Necessary?

Physical fitness is a factor in health and longevity but it is not the major factor. Recalling Dr de Lacy Evans' survey of people who lived for a hundred years or more, many of the centenarians were sedentary throughout their lives, and although their exercise habits, drinking habits and smoking habits varied widely, the one thing they displayed in common was that they had always partaken sparingly of food.

The degree of physical exercise needed by any individual to maintain good health depends primarily on the degree of physical fitness required for whatever tasks are required of them, and this standard will be automatically achieved as they become competent at the tasks. Above a reasonable level of fitness there is no added health advantage to be gained (bearing in mind the facts relating to heart disease, blood viscosity, etc) and if carried to extremes physical exercise can be highly stressful and counterproductive to the intended purpose.

The Role of Sunshine, Fresh Air and Rest

Sunshine and fresh air as health factors important to the restoration of sick people back to health have been well known for hundreds of years, and therefore no further discussion about them will be needed. It also goes without saying that rest should be adequate.

A full dissertation on the importance of direct natural sunlight and the benefits to be derived from not excessive exposure to natural ultraviolet light energy is given in the Chapter "Natural Light and Health" in *The Health Revolution*, if a deeper understanding of the physiology involved is desired.

Asthma

Asthma is the restriction of breathing caused by the swelling of the bronchial tubes through which air is inhaled in the lungs and carbon dioxide exhaled. The swelling is due to a toxic bloodstream and is exacerbated by emotional stress in the same way as other disease conditions are exacerbated when extra fatty acids enter the bloodstream. Irritation by airborne particles such as pollen may also exacerbate the condition but, like stress, is not the primary cause of the disease.

Asthma quickly clears once a very low-fat diet is adopted and the blood freed of lipotoxemia, and asthma is no exception to the rule—applicable to all diseases— that physical exercise is of similar benefit. Although less effective than diet, the effect of regular sustained exercise is to free the blood of fats and lower the blood viscosity. A typical example of the benefits of exercise is the report in the Australian *Woman's Day* on 31 December 1991. The article headed "I took the plunge and beat Asthma" described how a lady, thin and weak with asthma at age forty-five took up swimming on her doctor's advice and is now, at the age of fifty-nine, happy and healthy although still not completely free of asthma. She could be, if she dieted properly (*see* Chapter 16).

Arthritis (and Rheumatism)

Whereas arthritis is considered medically to be an auto-immune disease in which white blood cells supposedly attack the body's own tissues, it is nothing of the sort. There are two ways white cells become involved in the cause of arthritis:

1 When uric acid levels resultant of excessive protein intake become so high as to precipitate uric acid crystals in the joints, the white cells (phagocytes) endeavor to destroy the crystals but are instead themselves destroyed by the crystals, and their corrosive digestive juices which are effective against other antigens, but not uric acid, are liberated into the joints, damaging them.
2 In conditions of high blood viscosity due to lipotoxemia, oxygen levels in the synovial fluid of joints becomes so low that white cells in the area perish for want of it and their corrosive juices are, as in the uric acid case, liberated as the agent of joint damage.

Thus arthritis is caused by either excess protein or excess fat in the diet, or both, and is exacerbated by emotional stress which as a normal physiological event leads to the release of extra fatty acids into the blood. It should be noted that the high intake of vegetable protein and fats is as capable of producing arthritis as are animal protein and fats; and that it is a mistake to consume grain products, lentils, etc in the belief they are healthful.

In most cases relief from arthritis is achieved in a few days once proper dietary procedures are adopted.

Cancer

Toxemia again is the cause of this disease as has already been explained—excess fat, protein, cholesterol and salt being the main culprits together with deficiencies of fresh green vegetables and fruit. Emotional status has a great bearing on either accelerating or retarding the progress of cancer, as of course it does with any sickness.

There are many cases on record of "spontaneous remission" of cancer, when to the astonishment of doctors cancer mysteriously diminished and completely cleared. "Spontaneous remissions" are regarded as medical phenomena beyond comprehension, but it is obvious they are natural events achieved by the healing powers within the body when for some reason or other homeostasis has been regained.

Thus the immediate measures for cancer must be to eliminate from the lifestyle every single adverse factor leading to toxemia and to diminution of the immune system, and to instil confidence and determination with the goal of achieving a complete spontaneous remission. This advice should not be construed as medical advice; on the contrary, it is advice for reconstituting a healthy *milieu interieur*, the only basis upon which the reversal of cancer is possible (*see* Chapter 16). For a more detailed explanation of cancer read *The Health Revolution* by this author and *A Cancer Therapy, Results of Fifty Cases* by Dr Max Gerson.

"Spontaneous remissions" of cancer are more numerous than is commonly believed, as is recounted in *The Health Revolution*, and they would be more the rule rather than the exception if patients knew what to do and were confident enough to refuse the conventional treatment which has never been proven to prolong life.

For the achievement of recovery from cancer, the importance of a positive, determined attitude by the patient cannot be over-emphasized. Dr Paul Pearsall, in his book *Super Immunity* (Ebury Press, London, 1987), described the collection of 400 cases of spontaneous remissions and their review by Dr Elmer Green and his wife Dr Alyce Green, looking for explanatory factors. The one factor above all that was common in every case was that every one of the patients had changed their mental attitude to one of hope and were more positive about surviving. This point has already been covered in preceding pages but, once again, it cannnot be over-emphasized (*see* Alfred Keane's letter in Chapter 16).

Diabetes

As already explained in Chapter 6, in most cases the pancreas of people with diabetes is perfectly capable of producing the insulin needed for the metabolism of the body's blood sugar, in fact sometimes double the amount. The reason that diabetes occurs in the presence of adequate insulin is that an excess of blood fats (lipotoxemia) inhibits the insulin from interacting with the sugar, so that all that is needed to restore most diabetics to normal is to get rid of the fat out of their bloodstreams. It is not a coincidence that most diabetics are overweight. Diabetics suffer all sorts of circulatory problems including heart disease, hypertension, glaucoma, blindness and so on, not because they have diabetes but because of the lipotoxemia which is also the cause of their diabetes.

Thus while diabetics can be assisted to metabolize their blood sugar by injecting them with extra insulin over and above that which they are producing themselves, the underlying cause—lipotoxemia—remains. When it is "officially" stated that diabetes is a leading cause of death it is no such thing; the cause of death among diabetics is none other than lipotoxemia which also causes their glaucoma, blindness and other associated problems. This information, as previously mentioned, has been known, in detail, since 1936, and experiments in the 1960s demonstrated that fit young athletes could be made (temporarily) diabetic in two days simply by loading their food with fat and protein and, in fact even in two hours, if lipids (fats) were infused directly into their blood.

The Pritikin Center in Santa Monica has demonstrated for years that most diabetics can be taken completely off their medication in just a couple of weeks on a very low-fat and low-protein diet (*see The Health Revolution*), and it will also be recalled from Chapter 6 how diabetic city-dwelling Aboriginals quickly became free of diabetes when they are relocated on their tribal grounds where they resume their traditional native foods again.

Heart Disease, Stroke, Hypertension and other Circulatory Problems

It was shown in the 1960s that diseased arteries can clean and heal themselves when the blood is cleansed of lipotoxemia, and everybody knows that thin gravy is easier to pour than thick gravy, which means of course that thin blood is easier to pump around the body than sticky blood. Thus the greatest benefit someone can bestow on their body is to get rid of toxemia and unstick their blood. Straightaway the blood's function is improved while at the same time areas deprived of circulation regain it—one of which may be the heart muscle itself—so that the workload on the heart is lessened, the blood pressure lowered, and all systems improve, including vitality and mental acuity.

It is important to understand that the lowering of blood viscosity is vital in cases of restricted circulation, because doing so removes the patient from immediate danger. Thus somebody with almost totally blocked coronary (or other) arteries can often proceed with normal activities, even strenuous exercise, without discomfort because of the natural bypass provided by collateral circulation around the blocked sections. Collateral circulation is provided by the growth of a great number of fine capillary vessels, which is the body's attempt to overcome the local problem, and is completely effective provided the blood is thin enough to flow through the fine vessels. But should the blood viscosity increase as the result of blood fats released into the blood by way of a fatty meal, sudden stress, or vigorous exercise, the collateral circulation suddenly can no longer function and a heart attack ensues. There are thousands of coronary bypass operations conducted every day on people who already have natural bypasses capable of doing the job providing they avoid the things that thicken up their blood. The invention of the coronary bypass was a brilliant technological achievement, a boon to surgeons and a boon (often temporary) to people who are incapable of foregoing the dietary pleasures that caused their problem in the first place. As a coronary bypass can itself block up in as short a time as a year or two, it is essential in order to ensure survival that proper dietary measures are adopted anyway. In preference to undergoing major surgery, a far better course of action in most cases would be to emulate Rolet de Castella of Melbourne and others like him. Rolet, himself a coronary bypass candidate after a stroke in 1974 and a heart attack in 1975, opted for do-it-yourself natural therapy, starting with a severe dietary change which quickly gave him the capacity to resume his sport of long distance running and to abandon all his medication. Since then he has completed over thirty marathon races, all traces of his circulatory problems having long since passed entirely.

Osteoporosis

This has already been explained in a previous chapter, but to reiterate: osteoporosis is merely the natural reaction of the body trying to protect itself from the internal acidity caused by the intake of excessive protein, whereby calcium from the bones is sacrificed to neutralize the acid which, if not so neutralized, would cause even greater harm. Osteoporosis is therefore the lesser of two evils and completely avoidable by avoiding the excessive protein intake which is a feature of the modern diet equally contributory to toxemia as the excesses of fat and cholesterol.

Nephritis

As it is the function of the kidneys to filter out and excrete impurities from the blood, it is not surprising that people on the Western diet, heavily encumbered with toxemia, suffer a great deal of kidney trouble sometimes to the degree of complete kidney failure. Impurities, precipitated out of solution from the blood that the kidneys are unable to cope with, often build up to form stones in the kidneys composed of residues of uric acid and calcium. While conventional medical procedure is to physically remove kidney stones, once the body is freed of toxemia the stones, just like cholesterol build-ups in the arteries, gradually dissolve and disappear of their own accord.

Whereas the main dietary factor eventuating in kidney failure is the overconsumption of protein and condiments, more and more it is becoming evident that kidney failure is also frequently attributable to antibiotics and other medical drugs.

Gallstones

These are another feature distinguishing people who indulge heavily in animal protein foods. The arteries are not the only tissues that are forced to accept fat and cholesterol in excess of the body's capacity to excrete. In high concentrations cholesterol precipitates into crystals, and an indication of an enthusiastic meat-eater is the whitish ring around the iris of the eye consisting of cholesterol crystals (arcus senilus). It is of such crystals that gallstones are principally composed in the gallbladder, but again, like kidney stones, once the condition of toxemia is removed the gallstones gradually dissolve and disappear.

Mental Aberrations

As the brain in use consumes for its size a great deal more fuel (blood sugar) and oxygen than any other organ of the body, it is provided with a copious blood supply and, like any of the other organs, works best if the blood is pure and well oxygenated.

Nathan Pritikin described tests with children given a number of simple arithmetic sums to do, which showed that after a while on a very low-fat diet their mental performance both in speed and accuracy improved by twenty per cent. On the other end of the scale, senile people put on the same diet regained memory and control of body functions which beforehand they had lost. This being so, it is plain to see why the top levels in school examination results are so often gained by children of Oriental migrants who have yet to a adopt the Western diet, although a recent news item reports that it doesn't take long before the children of migrants soon adopt our dietary ways and at the same time begin to exhibit the physical deterioration that distinguishes our children.

With children at one end of the age scale and senile adults at the other, both groups demonstrating the diminished mental and physical standards that accompany a high-fat diet, it is a safe bet that just about everybody in the age groups in between are similarly affected, including of course our politicians, many of whom display disturbing signs of mental incapacity.

Fish is often referred to as a "brain food", but if that appears to be the case it would not be because fish contains some magical ingredient, but more because it is less likely than meat to make the blood sticky, which of course is the reason heart attacks occur with less frequency among the people in coastal fishing villages compared to farming villages not far distant inland.

When it is known that vegetarians display happier and more placid demeanors than meat-eaters, apart from better general health, it is clear that not only can drugs affect mental processes but so too can toxemia derived from food. Behavioral problems such as hyperactvity in children, emotional outbursts and schizophrenia in adults, can all be related to toxemia and lipotoxemia derived from diet, and it is only one step further to inquire what little extra influence from alcohol or some other drug, perhaps even just stress, does it need to turn some quiet man into one of the crazy gunmen you read about?

Constipation

Constipation, which is a major factor in the toxemia underlying most of the other common complaints, occurs for two reasons:

1 Wrong food containing too much fat and not enough vegetable fiber.
2 Incorrect posture for defecation. The natural posture for defecation is the squatting position. While standing or sitting there is a kink in the anal canal which is an effective seal which has to be overcome by extra pressure in order to expel the contents of the bowel; but when squatting the kink straightens out and the bowel movement is much easier. In Asian countries where toilet pans sit flush with the floor, and with the other advantages of a diet containing greater amounts of vegetables, constipation is not the universal problem it is in Western countries.

The adoption of the squatting position for defecation not only soon achieves freedom from constipation but solves also the problem of urinary incontinence in women[1] and relief of prostate disorders in men, while at the same time allowing the natural healing of hemorrhoids.

---

[1] Squatting is also the natural position for childbirth.

Thus it can be seen that when toxemia exists, every single function of the body is to some extent adversely affected, worsening as the years go by as the body's vital organs deteriorate and become less and less able to achieve homeostasis.

ME: Chronic Fatigue Syndrome, etc

Refer to the Afterword by Dr Gaye Keir in Chapter 16.

AIDS

There are a great many cases of arresting the condition of AIDS and regaining stabilized good health. There is a list of books written by AIDS survivors in the Appendix, but the procedure to restore the body from AIDS (or cancer) is no different than resolving any other health problem except perhaps for one thing: and that is first and foremost to reject and totally banish from the mind that AIDS (or cancer) is irreversible and fatal. Only the cases in which the immune system is completely shattered is this so.

The rules for recovery then are:

1 Think positive, others have done it, so can you. Remember, few doctors know the real facts about AIDS, they know only what they have accepted, parrot-fashion, from the incompetent American AIDS establishment.
2 Reject all medical treatment. In ten years and having used up billions of dollars in research funds unsuccessfully trying to prove the HIV theory of AIDS, the medical establishment has not saved *one* life of an AIDS patient, and this is not because AIDS is fatal; it is because the *medical procedures are fatal*.
3 Eliminate all drugs of any kind—even aspirin—from your life, forever, including of course nicotine.
4 Adopt the dietary procedures recommended in Chapter 14: no more junk food, salt, sugar.
5 Supplement the diet with a minimum of ten grams a day of vitamin C.

6 Get fit.
7 Get adequate sleep.
8 No excesses, sexual or otherwise.
9 Get plenty of fresh air and sunshine.
10 Instead of feeling sorry for yourself, go out and help somebody else, even if only to give them a smile.
11 Get your teeth fixed, but not with amalgam (mercury) fillings.
12 Others have done it, so can you. Remember, if a man thinks he can, or if he thinks he cannot, he's right either way.

Other diseases of civilization

Premenstrual tension, migraine, schizophrenia, premature senility, Alzheimer's disease, diminished mental acuity, failing eyesight, cataracts, diminished hearing, skin problems, ulcers, kidney stones, gallstones, varicose veins, estrogen imbalance, prostate inflammation, multiple sclerosis and so on, regardless of whatever 'high-tech' names are given them, can all be arrested and in most cases completely reversed, once the body's chemical imbalance has been corrected and homeostasis restored. The only cases in which the body is incapable of regaining homeostasis and achieving subsequent healing are those in which one or more vital organs have broken down irreparably, but because such complete failure is never a certainty, hope should never be abandoned even in the most advanced stages of degeneration. Even if organs are left with only a fraction of their original capacity, when the causes of toxemia are avoided the remaining capacity of the organ may still be sufficient to permit normal body functions. The recuperative powers of the body once homeostasis is restored are almost beyond belief.

CHAPTER 16

The Proof of the Pudding

by William Howard Hay MD
A chapter from Dr Hay's book *A New Health Era* (1933)

God does not perform his work so imperfectly or short-sightedly as to be obliged to interpose with miracles to set it right.

Leo H. Grindon
Lecturer on Botany, Royal School of Medicine
Manchester, 1860

"The writer is no magician or worker of miracles, neither does he claim the slightest credit for recovery in any case he accepts for treatment, for he realizes far more keenly than do most that recovery is a function of the body alone, and Nature, as represented by the body, has her own ways for repairing this useful automaton when out of order, and all any human being can do is to successfully interpret Nature and give her what assistance is possible in the way of removal of the visible handicaps to her work.

"He has the Scotch habit of insisting that two and two should always make four, and if otherwise then he is being gypped.

"It took fifteen years of patient and persistent application of the principles here laid out to remove finally and definitely from his so-called mind all specificity of disease, and to enable him to regard all disease as one thing, subject to the same rules and requiring the same form of treatment.

"To him now a toothache is merely an evidence of wrong chemical conditions of the body, conditions that he believes he can suggest as universal in all departures from health.

"Progressive pernicious anemia, asthma, Bright's disease, diabetes, rheumatism, arthritis, neuritis, gastric or duodenal ulcer, every form of digestive disturbance, eczema, psoriasis, pityriasis, goitres of all types, tumors, tuberculosis—any and all of these varied forms of so-called disease fall under one head, chemical imbalance of the body, and all subject to restoration to the normal through correction of the body chemistry and thorough drainage.

"This is a radical simplification of the consideration of disease, and takes this out of the realm of mystery.

"The very fact that all these varied conditions recover to a high normal is surely proof enough of the correctness of the theory, and it matters nothing that high authority says these things are wholly unmanageable by any known form of treatment.

"Such statement merely proves that the so-called authority does not know the cause of these conditions, therefore is not a good guide for anyone seeking relief.

"When the best that medical science can do for any of the conditions mentioned above is to temporize and treat symptoms and recognize them all as incurable, surely there must be something wrong with their ideas of the origin of any of them and how to correct this.

"To regard disease as merely a departure from normal health, no matter what form this departure takes, simplifies its consideration so greatly that it does not require medical training to appreciate it fully, nor anything resembling talent to find means for its relief, as the understanding of the thing carries automatically with it the knowledge of how to return to health.

"It was said earlier that all we can do for disease is to stop creating this background of acid end-products of digestion and metabolism, and this is true, for if disease comes always and only from this acid collection, then it must be evident to anyone that the cure lies in the discontinuance of this accumulation.

"Septic troubles of all kinds yield to simple detoxication and dietary correction wholly without sera or drugs or anything else.

"In deep types of blood poisoning the use of three heaping tablespoonsful of Epsom or Glauber salts, or a half pint of concentrated Pluto water, on an empty stomach, repeated if necessary for three or more days, and with diet of nothing but water, or surely nothing more than orange juice or other unsweetened juice, has not to this very date failed to restore the body to a near enough normal so that the temperature has subsided, and appetite has returned, usually within two or three days, even after antistreptococcic serum had been used and many forms of medication, without regulation of the diet or detoxication by purging.

"Temperature ranging up to 105°F [40.5°C], with chills, delirium, collapse, the count of the white cells enormous, have after two to three days shown normal temperature, have rapidly come back to normal, and showed a very high degree of health afterward, with no sequelae remaining to tell of the stresses of the past two weeks.

"Pneumonia, erysipelas, typhoid fever, influenza, acute arthritis, colitis, hay fever, all subside when the body is fairly detoxicated and the diet so corrected as to stop this excessive formation of the acid end-products, simply because each was expressing the end-point of tolerance of toxins, and each was the means by which the body sought to unload this unwanted mass.

"The acute fevers of little children pass in one night, as a rule, leaving the little one wanting food the very next day, and no matter how small the child this crisis meant always the same thing, which was that the little body had accumulated toxins to the point of tolerance and was now trying to unload them by means of a fever, or heightened oxidation process, during which much of this waste is burned and thrown out.

"Little children can scarcely be made to take the nauseating dose of salts or Pluto water, so the tasteless castor oil is better here, using double the prescribed dose in every case.

"The object of the purge is not the movement of the bowels, though this is accomplished also, but it is intended to remove from the body much of its acid-laden fluids, the serum from the blood, the lymph from the tissues.

"In the adult the use of a half pint of concentrated Pluto water will usually result in the ejection from the bowel of three or four quarts of fluid, and the thirst resulting from this dehydration will make the free use of fruit juices very gratifying. Thus an alkaline or base-forming source of supply is opened up for the body to replenish its deficient stores, and the condition of the body immediately is one of lowered acidity, or rather a heightened alkalinity.

'This is neutralizing much of the mass of acid end-products, hence the feeling of relief that usually follows this rather drastic purging, and the more toxic the condition the greater the feeling of relief.

"Many cases of nephritis, with broken heart compensation, unable to walk about through weakness, unable to lie down because of the shortness of breath, will purge for three days and then lie down flat to sleep and even take walks with enjoyment, and all without any food whatever.

"Always before coming under treatment an effort had been made to 'keep up the strength' with foods of all sorts, and yet in spite of this free feeding they were extremely weak, but after this spasm of intensive detoxication they were stronger at once, without food.

"This would seem to indicate that the weakness formerly was from the intoxication, and the relief of this by the drastic purge allowed of better function at once, accounting for the seeming increase in strength, and surely there seems to be no other way to look at it.

"Nephritis, or Bright's disease as it is usually called, is one of the very deep types of intoxication, and what is accomplished there is duplicated by the beforementioned blood infections, as streptococcic infection, or so-called blood poisoning, where the immediate relief from the purge and fast or near-fast, is rather impressive, especially to one who is familiar with the usual course of these unmanageable conditions.

"True anginas, whether from degenerative changes in the heart muscle or from embolism of the coronary artery, will generally lose all pain on exertion after three days of active purging and fruit juice diet, and go on to complete relief, even returning to active exercise, golf, even tennis, and with no remaining evidence of heart incompetency.

"Every case of arthritis short of actual anchylosis, or fixation of joints, will respond to treatment, and complete recovery is the rule, not the exception, the result limited only by the degree of fixation of the joints.

"Many a case of gastric or duodenal ulcer responds at once, the very first day of fruit juices bringing grateful relief, but in those cases of bleeding ulcer it is not wise to use the drastic purge to start the detoxication period, for fear of exciting haemorrhage.

"It is enough to empty the colon daily by means of the simple enema and confine the food wholly to the fruit juices till all pain has completely subsided, then begin feeding with the wholly alkaline foods, as cooked vegetables, raw vegetable salads, fresh fruits, and a moderate amount of milk or buttermilk, the latter preferred.

"To date no case of gastric or duodenal ulcer has failed to entirely recover, though some go through several recurrences, usually each lighter and shorter than preceding attacks; but the thing is cyclic in character, and tends to return at intervals of six months to one year, a few cases having cycles of two years, when the attack comes on, is severe for a time, then gradually subsides, no one knows why; but it is thinkable that the pain of digestion so limits the intake of food that in time there is relief from the irritation that produces the trouble. If it were not for the fact that the victim when relieved of pain returns to his former incompatible habits of eating he would not suffer recurrences, but when the history is long, and there have been many cycles, the cause is so deeply rooted that even correct eating may not be sufficient to guarantee freedom from recurrences till the body's chemistry is well changed. However, each case recovers ultimately, proving that a hyper-acid state of the body was the cause, for only alkalinization of the body was required for cure.

"The late Dr Sippy, of Chicago, who specialized in the treatment of gastric and duodenal ulcer for many years, made the statement on the floor of the Erie County Medical Society not long before his death, that every case of gastric or duodenal ulcer was originally a hyperchlorhydria, meaning that a too free production of hydrochloric acid in the gastric juice was the active irritant in every case.

"The writer's experience fully bears out this statement of Dr Sippy, but the so-called Sippy diet, or bland diet, while it does give relief, never ultimately cures, for there is always a tendency to recurrence of the cycles till the whole body chemistry is changed to a more alkaline state, a thing Dr Sippy did not believe. Hence his cases returned to him again and again with recurrences, while if the diet had been sufficiently alkaline throughout, very few cases would have ever suffered relapse, and in time all cases would have recovered permanently.

"The word 'permanently' is used advisedly, though it carries with it the understanding that a repetition of the former wrong habits of eating would insure a return of the ulcer.

"One hundred and nine cases of progressive pernicious or primary anemia passed through the same simple form of detoxication and dietary correction, and all but eight recovered, the eight simply being too far gone to permit of time for the necessary changes.

"In every recovery the result was permanent except in those who returned to careless habit of diet and neglected to thoroughly empty the colon every day.

"Of course a repetition of the original causes would naturally tend to produce the same result, as the original attack showed the weak link in the chain of resistance, and a similar toxic condition would be quite likely to express through this same weak point.

"Primary or progressive pernicious anemia is a failure of the blood making organs, as against a secondary anemia, which is due to destruction of the red cells from some internal or external toxic material, and the secondary type disappears when this source of destruction is found and corrected.

"The primary type has been long considered a mystery, and no one attempted to tell the origin of the influence that depressed the function of the blood making organs.

"The chronic asthmatic, the spasmodic type, is probably the most grateful and the most greatly surprised of all chronic sufferers, for usually he has been everywhere, has tried everything, has consulted the best specialists, and has been told everywhere that nothing can be done for him except to send him to a higher and dryer climate, and usually this also is found to give but little and temporary relief.

"The very first week, in the majority of cases, shows marked relief from spasm, and in the case of young children even a week is more than is necessary to show this, for many of them never again have the slightest sign of asthma after even less than a week following three days of drastic purging and alkaline diet.

"The relief seems to the asthmatic almost unbelievable, and it is not well to promise such speedy relief in the beginning, for this sufferer has gone through too much to believe easily that his trouble of years past has been all this time such a simple thing, and then, too, his may be one case that requires a longer time, as some rare cases do.

"So the asthmatic is told that his case is curable if he will follow faithfully the directions given, and if he is one of the lucky ones and loses his whole trouble in the first few weeks of treatment he will be the happiest man in the world.

"Spasmodic or catarrhal asthma is nothing but a toxic state expressing through bronchial tubes that are not any too large at best, and it does not require much swelling of these little capillary tubes to seriously interfere with their function of carrying air into the lungs and carbonic acid gas out, so the victim smothers from this difficulty.

"As the hyper-acid state subsides so does the catarrhal swelling everywhere, and a little subsidence in the tiny bronchial tubes does make a great deal of difference in the breathing of anyone.

"It is not long ago that we began to recognize colitis as the frequent occurrence that it really is, and now we understand that every case of constipation is a colitis of degree, whether mucus is thrown off or not. Colitis is now regarded as so common that in almost every case presenting for treatment there will be found evidence of catarrh of the colon in some degree, just as we expect that few people will be able to say that they have the natural three bowel movements daily.

"If mucus is not observed in the stools it soon will be after the beginning of daily enemata and the correction of the diet to a more alkaline standard, and this first appearance usually leads the patient to think that the enema or the diet is doing harm, but the opposite is the case. The body is only beginning to unload this waste material, and the more mucus the better the indication, for this is accentuated elimination, and should go on till no more mucus is left to show in the stools.

"Colitis comes from the character of the contents of this neglected organ; a toxic mass, putrefying, fermenting, is retained too long, and unless the colon is emptied daily there will continue to be absorption from this sewer, and recovery will be delayed till it is borne in on the patient's mind that it is better to get this material out than to let it remain to further putrefy and ferment.

"There is not the slightest chance of permanently injuring the function of this organ by doing its work vicariously for a time, because its function depends on internal cleanliness as much as on anything else, though ultimate recovery of normal bowel tone is a matter of general revitalization of the whole body, and till this has had time to occur it will be necessary to continue to aid this burdened organ in this way.

"Every case of colitis recovers if the diet is correct and if the colon contents are daily flushed out by the simple enema till such time as returning general vitality restores the tone of every organ and part of the body, a period that varies from a few weeks to a few months in most cases, but in constipation of deep type and long history it may require two, three or more years to regain a competent activity of the colon.

"Next to constipation the common cold is perhaps the thing most prescribed for and least understood.

"The P.H.S. undertook an intensive study of colds some time ago, I believe at the suggestion of the president, but that this will accomplish anything is too much to expect, for there is little or nothing known about the real cause of this very common condition.

"The cold will never be properly understood till we realize that each attack is merely the body's end-point of tolerance for the acids of digestion and metabolism, and when we have ceased to create these toxic materials we will cease to manifest the common cold.

"When patients have kept the colon well up to the minute and have so corrected their dietary habit as to stop this excessive formation of adventitious acids, no more colds manifest, and in a few years no possible exposure can again produce this manifestation that we call a cold. Were this not true then everything before said would fall flat, for here is a very good way to prove the whole thing, and one would not dare to make any such statement as that colds will become impossible when the body has raised its alkalinity to anywhere near the normal, unless able to prove it.

"Eat all foods compatibly and bring the colon up to date and you will furnish yourself with all the proof necessary that it becomes impossible for you to 'catch cold'.

"Colds are not caught, they are accumulated with the feet under the dinner table, and in no other way.

"If you will stop creating the usual acid excesses and keep the colon up to date you will find plenty of other reasons to point to the general fact that disease of every sort comes from accumulation of these acid end-product of digestion and metabolism, and you will be abundantly impressed with the proof of all of the foregoing, and will begin to realize that after all old Mother Nature is your very best friend.

"You have not listened to her in the past or you would have long ago discover this, but start right in today to listen hard to all her suggestions, and you will come to have the most profound respect for her.

"It has often been said that Nature is a very good nurse, but a poor physician, and this is true enough, if by physician you mean one who treats disease, for she does not treat disease, and neither should we.

"We should ignore disease and concentrate on building health, which means that we should not fail to observe all the natural indications of the body in health or its opposite, and satisfy ourselves with keeping the laws of our own nutrition, and we will need only a nurse, and Nature is after all the very best.

"Sir William Osler once said that anything that cannot be cured by Nature must forever remain uncured, which would seem to indicate that he considered the old lady not only the best of nurses, but not so bad as a physician also.

"It is safe to say that of all the thousands of cases that have presented here for the past twenty-five years, by far the largest number were those who had gone through almost every form of so-called treatment at the hands of many physicians, but who, like the poor woman in the Bible, had spent all their substance, and grew nothing better, but rather grew worse. With few exceptions these have regained their lost health in part or in whole, and at the same time have learned the blessed lesson that as we eat so are we, and have been able since to conform sufficiently to the body's laws as to guarantee their health for the future.

"It is good to recover from supposedly unmanageable disease, but it is better, in a far larger way, to know why one has been less than well and just how to conserve the health and vitality for the future.

"This I consider constructive therapeutics; nothing else is, and till official medicine takes similar ground they should not complain if the public is losing confidence in their treatment of disease, and is turning to Osteopaths and Chiropractors, or even to Christian Science, the last abjuring all forms of treatment."

In regard to cancer, Dr Hay had this to say:

"As cancer is a systemic affair, expressing as a local growth, the removal of this evidence of cancer does not correct the system. Again the cart has been placed before the horse, in the prevalent belief that the local growth makes the systemic symptoms that accompany cancer, when as a matter of fact, the cancer condition exists long before there is a local expression of this in the form of growth or ulceration.

Yes, if cancer is of sufficiently slow growth it can be cured by fasting and proper diet though there must be time enough to allow the body to make a complete chemical re-adjustment, and many cases of cancer are recorded as cured by these simple means."

Further on Cancer and "The Doctor Within"

Perth
30th October 1991

Ross, I prefer to call you by your given name because I feel that you are a very special person and I feel as many others would, very much in debt to you.

I will not bore you with the details of how I was notified (after six months) that I had prostate cancer, and by the time they found that out I had bone cancer too and the shocking wasting disease that took all my flesh away. I was told to go home as there was nothing they could do to help me.

I went home, but on the way out fate had put a man

sitting on the edge of his bed. He said to me, "I am sorry to hear of your bad news." I am sixty-nine and I said to him, "Well, we have three score years and ten so I guess after what I have just been told I have one left, a year that is." Actually, I had three to four months according to the medical panel who had dealt with me. He said, "BULLSHIT! You are too young and fit to die." He added, "Cancer is a word, not a sentence."

He told me about you. I was told to buy *The Health Revolution*, fourth edition, and read it over and over.

Then he told me to contact a Mr Garth Squires at Bullsbrook, who was a friend of yours, and at one time had been only days away from dying of cancer himself.

Garth gave me detailed instructions of what I must do.

I went home that night and my son nursed me all night and I cried in his arms as the pain and worry took over. Your book was in short supply but I got a copy and never have I read a book so avidly as I did this one. I started the Gerson diet straight away. I have remained on raw fresh fruit since that day. I beat the pain bit by bit but it was tough and awful.

I lost 3½ stone [22 kg] of the 9 stone [57 kg] that I weighed when this started. I am of small build: 5′6″ [1.6 m]. I looked like I had just stepped out of a POW camp—all bones. I stayed static for six weeks, then in two months I have put on 10 lb [4½ kg]. All pain has gone, the bladder is functioning, all my current crop of skin cancers fell off plus some nasty lumps on my body.

A blocked nerve channel is clean. New discs have grown in my neck (three were out according to my doctor, whom I may add won't have anything to do with me. Strange!).

It is a miracle. I have faith. I do not know why people are so blind.

Nature's food as God intended us to eat is all there, my body is restoring itself more each day, I can even hear the phone ring and that's the first time in ten years.

There is a bit of a story there Ross: Garth told me to write to you and relate it.

I can only say that the information I gleaned from your wonderful book put me on the right track. Garth Squires has been a boon to me when I lost hope.

All this story has evolved over a period of six months. My blood pressure is normal and all systems are go.

I thank you Ross Horne that you are all the things that you are. I thank you for your brilliance in what you have achieved and may you continue a long and active life in those achievements.

Yours most faithfully,
Alfred Keane

Afterword on Chronic Fatigue Syndrome

(by Dr Gaye Keir, Brisbane)

"In late 1984 I was perusing the books in my local bookstore when I came across a copy of Ross Horne's *The Health Revolution*. It looked interesting, so I bought it to add to my collection of health-oriented books—a collection which existed for both professional and personal reasons. Professional because I was a psychologist interested in the relationship between health and lifestyle factors. Personal because I was being faced with an ever-increasing number of my own health problems, in spite of what I believed was a healthy lifestyle—aerobic exercise, meditation, and carefully selected food.

"For years I had suffered on and off with a variety of complaints—head and chest colds, bronchitis, recurrent sore throats, headaches, back pain, leg cramps, generalised muscular pain, chronic conjunctivitis, sensitivity to light, 'cold' attacks, menstrual abnormalities, weight fluctuations, acne, skin complaints, 'crawling' sensations, tinnitus, loss of hearing. The worst complaint of all and the one which in the end sent me so relentlessly in search of a cure was a chronic lack of energy, which in the final months

before changing my diet left me sleeping anywhere between
ten and fifteen hours a day. During my waking hours I
could barely drag myself around and had no motivation
to attack even the simplest task.

"In December 1985, my health reached crisis point
and I sought a medical opinion about my deteriorating
state. The doctors I saw (a general practitioner and four
specialists) authorised extensive tests—including tests for
diabetes and hypothyroidism, a brain scan, and vestibular
function tests. With the exception of one test, I proved
completely 'normal'. (The exception was that an audio-
gram suggested some nerve and middle ear cell damage
in the right ear, thus accounting for my hearing loss and
tinnitus.)

"Most of the doctors came to the same conclusion—
I was depressed or psychologically stressed in some way
and I would be best helped by seeing a psychiatrist. I resisted
this suggestion most strongly. I have worked in psychology
most of my adult life—I obtained a doctorate in 1977 and
I worked for several years as an academic. I was convinced
that psychological problems were not the cause of my poor
health and my chronic lack of energy.

"By then I had started reading books about food
sensitivities, and was aware that my pattern of symptoms
was consistent with such a problem. So having satisfied
myself that there was nothing 'medically' wrong with me,
and refusing to believe that my problems were
psychological, I started to look at the effect of the food
I was eating.

"I took *The Health Revolution* off my shelf and started
reading it in earnest. It was a book which I was to find
fascinating but startling in its advocation of a fruitarian
diet. I already knew something of the Pritikin program
and had even changed my diet in the direction of reducing
my animal protein and oil intake. But I was struggling
with my conventional ideas about nutrition—the necessity
for a 'varied' diet, the need for some animal protein for
B_{12}, dairy products for calcium. I had been seduced for
so long by that false argument of nutrition—that because

a food contains a particular nutrient that we need, then that food must be good for us.

"In the beginning I thought that maybe I just had 'food sensitivities', so one by one I started eliminating foods from my diet. Virtually the first to go was grains—an elimination which caused me great difficulty since grains had previously been the highlight of my meals. My addiction to them was very strong, and I would literally go in search of them if they were not available.

"Over a period of several weeks, I eliminated specific food groups—grains, animal protein, nuts and seeds, tea and coffee, oil and fats. Through a process of elimination, all that was left were fruit and vegetables. Almost immediately I noticed a dramatic improvement in my energy levels and my overall health. I also noticed that the more fruit I ate and the less of everything else, the better I felt. At the same time I was reading and rereading *The Health Revolution*. Slowly, I was becoming convinced—from both a logical and an empirical point of view—that the answer was not to eliminate foods to which I was sensitive, but to choose a diet that would give me optimal health.

"Two years on—April 1988—I am still largely fruitarian. My diet consists mainly of a variety of fresh fruit (including avocado) and some fresh vegetables, usually eaten raw. During the past two years my health has been excellent. I have not had a cold or bronchitis in all that time and almost without exception all my other symptoms have disappeared, including my lack of energy. I currently work between fifty and sixty-five hours a week, as well as maintaining a mild but regular exercise program.

"Recent blood tests show that my biochemistry is normal and that I have a normal blood count. My triglycerides are low— 0.7 mmol/l—thus discounting Nathan Pritikin's fear that a large intake of fruit would lead to increased triglyceride levels. Bone density tests show that I have an above average density for my age. So not only does my own health attest to the positive benefits of the fruit diet, but also standard medical tests demonstrate that I am not lacking any nutrients.

"There have been times when I have tried to re-introduce other foods into my diet—particularly grains—and always without success. Initially, there is little problem. But as I persist, one by one my old symptoms start to reappear—muscular pain, skin problems and fatigue are generally the first to surface. I have no choice but to revert to the fruit and vegetable routine.

"I do not believe that my recovery can be explained away as a placebo effect. My ill-health was too long standing and too diverse. My recovery too complete. Nor do I believe that I just suddenly stopped getting sick. My poor health was progressing slowly but surely in spite of consistent attempts on my part to lead a healthy lifestyle. And no other positive change occurred in my life at the same time as I changed my diet. So there was nothing else to explain the improvement.

"My expectations of fruitarianism were certainly not greater than my expectations of aerobic exercise, meditation and other diets. To be honest, my expectations of fruitarianism were extremely cautious, having experienced limited success in the past with my other programmes. And I can reproduce my symptoms any time I like—just by breaking the diet. Personally I would much prefer a more variable diet to be possible. Having eaten 'regular' food for most of my life, each day presents a challenge to cope with my addiction to it and not to succumb to all the sights and smells. I have no doubt that if I want good health, I have no choice."

A Story from the Heart

Queensland
18th March 1992

Dear Ross,
I don't want to bore you with a long story but I came out of Prince Charles Hospital, Brisbane, just after Christmas. I had been sent there by a specialist for open

heart surgery but after they took an Echo-gram, they decided that my heart was just too bad to do anything. I was fine tuned on to some drugs and sent home with the doctor's departing handshake and "We shall be seeing you again— I expect."

Life, though not so bad as some of your readers, was for me pretty poor. I couldn't stand up without blacking out—I had to sleep sitting up and couldn't walk further than 200 yards and that very slowly, without sitting down for a rest—and often needing an anginine tablet to get me back home.

I am a retired RAF pilot that's getting on a bit. I flew through WW2, the Berlin Air Lift, the Malayan Campaign and the Korean War—mostly in Sunderlands— then on to exploding the A and H bombs—22 years of flying. So when I heard that a QANTAS pilot had written *The Health Revolution*, I took the trouble to get a copy of the book and read it. I was so fit at the time (ie my wife and I had just sailed our 30ft catamaran out here from England) that I really didn't take a lot of notice of what I was reading—after all, I was already on a Weight Watcher's diet at the time. So you can imagine how shocked I was when they told me in hospital that the terrible chest pain was a heart attack, and that was nearly two years ago. Since then we have been back to the UK and travelled 10,000 miles over the British Isles but on my return home here, I had another attack—and finished up in Prince Charles Hospital.

This time, when I came out of hospital, my wife said: "Right, we go to the library and see if Ross Horne has brought out any new books." This we did and found you had.

I read *Improving on Pritikin* from cover to cover (plus re-reading *The Health Revolution* again) and found your arguments water tight. I immediately went on to the full fruit and raw vegetable diet, except that I still have the need of a cup of tea, two or three times a day (made with no sugar and skim milk).

Ross, I can hardly believe the improvement in my

heart. After only three weeks I am walking two miles, can stand up to attention and salute without blacking out and at night I am sleeping like a baby on my back flat. I am afraid to talk about it as I am very superstitious and I am scared I might have a set-back. But I feel I must thank you for producing this book, which has changed my poor life to an exciting one again. The amount of research and sheer hard work which you must have put into this book is very much appreciated. I drive my car and nip around (with some caution) like a 40 year old, and am making plans to visit the UK next year (via QANTAS—who else?).

I have already bought three copies of your book, which I have passed on to relatives and friends—and have ordered another three more.

I wish you every success and very good health. If by chance you are ever planning to give lectures anywhere on the Sunshine Coast, my wife and I would deem it a privilege to attend. Please let us know if you have been able to open a type of Longevity Centre in Australia— if so could you let us know more about it.

Very kind regards,
Sincerely,
B.C. Horsnell, Sqn Ldr RAF Retd

Author's Note
I could fill a whole book with stories like these, but if I haven't got my point across by now, I never will.

However, if they give needed encouragement, more can be found in the chapter "Living Proof" in *The Health Revolution* and also in *Improving on Pritikin*. These include cases of recovery from MS, rheumatoid arthritis, hairy cell leukemia and, of course, cancer and heart disease.

CHAPTER 17

Epilogue

The history of mankind is an immense sea of errors in which a few obscure truths may here and there be found.

Cesare Beccaria

In the preceding chapters we have reviewed, at least in part, our immense sea of errors, and from it have extracted a few of the obscure truths, and have hopefully rendered those truths a little less obscure. To "straighten up and fly right", as Nat Cole would say, you need truths and not too many errors.

In regard to human relations, the 20th Century has produced its fair share of errors—wars, crime, ineptitude and so on, but on the credit side there have been some positive achievements such as women's emancipation, better understanding between nations, lessened racial and religious bigotry, recognition of environmental issues and so forth . . . not too bad an effort. Perhaps it could even be claimed that human intelligence has advanced a notch, although of course you could argue that point.

Now that the danger of World War III has passed, and aside from the global issues of overpopulation, environment, etc, the main threat to human existence today—as much in the developed countries as in the undeveloped—is the deterioration of peoples' health, together with the almost universal ignorance and indifference to that problem. The 21st Century could, if we played our cards right, produce a new Golden Age for mankind; but that will not happen because we have yet to learn how to play our cards right. Trial and error takes time.

There can be no Golden Age in a civilization beset with health problems and which does nothing about those problems other than to increase taxes to pay for drugs that only make things worse.

Louis Armstrong used to sing: "If it's good, then I want it, and if it's bad then I don't need it." The Russians, after seventy years of Communism, decided Communism was bad and they didn't need it, so they abandoned it— although only after it had just about completely ruined them . . .

The diseases of civilization pandemic in the Western world threaten to ruin everybody, while modern medicine is powerless to stop them. For instance, the death rate from heart disease and cancer currently in the USA is just on one and a half million every year which, in one year mind you, is five times the total number of US servicemen killed in battle in the entire four years of US participation in World War II. And modern scientific medicine can do nothing about it.

Like Communism, now abandoned by the Russians, "scientific" medicine has proven to be a failure and therefore so too is the "health-care" system that is designed around it, in the fallacious belief that health can be restored into a sick body by the administering of drugs. At least Communism works in theory if not in practice, but our health-care system is wrong both in theory *and* in practice, and only goes to prove the law of diminishing returns: the more you put into it, the more useless it becomes. A medical system that thrives on ill-health is an expensive millstone we cannot afford to carry, and if not soon curbed it will lead us into bankruptcy. Medical dogma with its empty promises is no better than Communist dogma and *its* empty promises so, as with Communism, the time has come to abandon it.

It has too long been mistakenly believed that technology will bring about a Golden Age, but this belief has been proven wrong because here at the end of the 20th

Century we are up to our ears in technology, but we are not as happy as we were fifty years ago. A golden age is an age of enlightenment, and for most of this century we have had the cart ahead of the horse; racing ahead with technology without the enlightenment to give it value.

But there is a change in the wind, a stirring of awareness, and there are signs that a new era of enlightenment has begun. In regard to health matters, perhaps Dr Alexis Carrel's prediction of 1936 has started to come true: "Unless the doctors of today become the dieticians of tomorrow, the dieticians of today will become the doctors of tomorrow." But time is running out. "Right now," says Dr Dean Burk (see foreword), "we are on dangerous ground, and whichever way we take there will be some rough going. *As ever, the fittest will survive.*"

Happy Landings

Book List of Recommended Reading

NOTE: Although the book list is divided under three headings: General, Cancer and AIDS, it should be remembered that all disease states are linked to unbalanced homeostasis one way or another, so that whatever a person's particular health problem may be, and whatever set of circumstances may have brought it about, the principles involved in restoring homeostasis will be the same in all cases. Thus there should be no attempt to search for specialised information once the required understanding of any single health problem has been gained. What I am trying to say is that you would not be wasting time if you read all the books.

Broadly, the books fall into three categories:

1 Those written by highly experienced doctors.
2 Those written by grateful survivors (some of them doctors).
3 Those written by investigative journalists.

Books marked with an asterisk are considered to be especially informative.

Many of the books are out of print and hard to locate. Two possible sources are Health Research, Mokelumne

Hill, California, and The Cancer Control Society, 2043 N. Berendo, Los Angeles.

To gain a deeper understanding of the processes that go on within the body, one has to become acquainted with the study of the Earth itself, the soil, the microbes in the soil, the plants, biology, physiology, anatomy and so on. Life and the nutrition that sustains it is an interesting and complex affair, which to find out if you've got it right you have to live 150 years! As far as I know the only people who have achieved this are simple peasants who aren't even interested! It's worth a try anyway . . .

General

Dissent in Medicine: Nine Doctors Speak Out, Robert Mendelsohn MD, George Crile MD, Samuel Epstein MD, Henry Heinlich MD, Alan Levin MD, Edward Pickney MD, David Spodick MD, Richard Moskowitz MD, Gregory White MD (Contemporary Books, 1985)

The Doctors, A Penetrating Analysis of the American Physician, Martin Gross (Random House, 1966)

Confessions of a Medical Heretic*, Dr Robert Mendelsohn (Contemporary Books, 1979)

Medicine Out of Control, The Anatomy of a Malignant Technology, Richard Taylor (Sunbooks, Melbourne, 1979)

What the Medical Establishment Won't Tell You That Could Save Your Life, Michael Culbert, Ph.D (Downing Publishers, Norfolk, Vancouver, 1983)

Medical Nemesis, Ivan Illich (Pantheon Press, 1975)

Limits of Medicine, Ivan Illich (Lothian Publishing, 1976)

The Body is the Hero, Dr Ronald Glasser (William Collins, 1977)

The Naked Empress or The Great Medical Fraud, Hans Ruesch (Buchverlag, CIVIS Publications, 1982)

The Great Billion Dollar Medical Swindle, Keith Lasks, MD (Bobbs-Merrill, Indianapolis, 1980)

Some Doctors Make You Sick. The Scandal of Medical Incompetence, Stephen Rice, BA, BL (Angus & Robertson, 1988)

Don't Call a Doctor, John Kerr (Veritas Publishing, Australia, 1987)

Health Shock, A Guide to Ineffective and Hazardous Medical Treatment, Martin Weitz (Reed Publishers, Sydney, 1980)

The Drug Story, Morris Beale (Biworld Publishers, Utah, 1949)

Pills That Don't Work, Sidney Wolfe, MD (Public Citizens Health Research Group, 1981)

Medical Drugs on Trial, Verdict Guilty, Kiki Sidhwa (Natural Hygiene Press, 1976)

Prescription Drugs, Peggy Mullen, Pharm.D (Beekman House, 1985)

Non-Prescription Drugs & Their Side Effects, Robert Benowicz (Grosset & Dunlop, 1977)

Prescription Drugs & Their Side Effects, Edward Stern (Putnam Publishing, NY, 1975-87)

The Drug Story, Morris Bealle (Biworld Publishers, 1949, 1976)

Vaccination Condemned, E. McBean, Ph.D (Better Life Research, Los Angeles, 1981)

The Solid Gold Stethoscope, Edgar Berman, MD (Macmillan, 1976)

Fluoridation, the Great Dilemma, Dr George Waldbott (Coronado Press, 1978)

Murder By Injection, Eustace Mullins (The National Council for Medical Research, Straunton, Vancouver, 1988)

Poison By Prescription. The AZT Story, John Lauritsen (Asklepois, New York, 1990)

A New Bacteriology, Drs Soren Sonea and Maurice Panisset (Jones & Bartlett, Boston, 1983)

Pasteur or Beauchamp?*, E. Douglas Hume (C.W. Daniel Co. 1923, Reprint 1989, Health Research)

The Genesis and Control of Disease*, Dr George Weger, MD (Phillips, Los Angeles, 1931)

The True Science of Living*, Dr Edward Dewey (Haskell & Son, London, 1899)

Human Life: Its Philosophy and Laws*, Dr Herbert Shelton (Health Research, Mokelumne Hill, California)

Impaired Health Cause and Cure*, Dr John Tilden, MD (Health Research)

Vitality, Fasting & Nutrition*, Dr Hereward Carrington, Ph.D (Health Research, Mokelumne Hill, California)

The Missing Link in the Medical Curriculum, Jay M. Hoffman, Ph.D (Professional Press)

Nutrition Health and Disease, Gary Todd, MD (Downing Publishers, 1985)

McDougall's Medicine, A Challenging Second Opinion, John McDougall, MD (New Century Publishers, 1985)

Old Age Deferred, Arnold Lorand, MD (F.A. Davis Co., Philadelphia, 1911)

Enzyme Nutrition*, Dr Edward Howell (Avery Publishing, Wayne, NJ, 1985)

Health and Long Life, Dr Bernard Jensen (Ommi Publishers, Escondido, Ca., 1975)

Primal Health, A Blueprint for Our Survival, Michael Odent, Surgeon (Century Hutchinson, 1986)

Immune For Life, Dr Arnold Fox (Medallion, 1986)

The New Science of Healing*, Dr Louis Kuhne (from the German) (Williams and Norgate, London, 1894)

The Low Fat Way to Health and Longer Life, Dr Lester Morrison (Prentice Hall, 1958)

What Your Doctor Didn't Learn in Medical School, Dr Stuart Berger (Bantam, 1988)

The Health Secrets of a Naturopathic Doctor, Dr Max Garten (Parker Publishing, New York, 1967)

A New Health Era*, Dr William Howard Hay (Pacono Hay-Ven, Mt Pocono, Pa., 1933)

Pottenger's Cats: A Study in Nutrition, Francis Pottenger, MD (Price-Pottenger Foundation, La Mesa, Ca., 1983)

The Prevention of the Diseases Peculiar to Civilization* (1929), Dr Sir William Arbuthnot Lane

Toxemia Explained*, Dr John Tilden (Health Research, 1927, 1952)

*The Health Handbook**, Dr Are Waerland, Ph.D (from the Swedish) (Humata Publications, Bern)

The Stress of Life, Hans Selye, MD (McGraw-Hill, 1956)

*How Nature Cures**, Dr Emmet Densmore (Stillman & Co, New York, 1892)

*How to Prolong Life**, Dr Charles DeLacy Evans, Ph.D (Charles Sawyer, London, 1910)

*The Wheel of Health**, Dr G.T. Wrench (C.W. Daniel Co, London, 1938)

*Sea Energy Agriculture**, Dr Maynard Murray (Valentine Books, Winston-Salem, NC, 1976)

*Man the Unknown**, Dr Alexis Carrel (Hamish Hamilton, London, 1935)

*The Wisdom of the Body**, Dr Walter Cannon (W.W. Norton, 1932)

*Nutrition and Physical Degeneration**, Weston Price, MSS DDS FACD (Price Pottenger Foundation, La Mesa, 1945)

The Diseases of Civilization, Brian Inglis, Ph.D (Granada, 1983)

*Human Degeneracy: Its Nature and Remedy**, Isaac Jennings, MD (Miller, Wood, New York, 1967)

Recovery From All Diseases, Masaharu Taniguchi, Ph.D (Seicho-No-Ie Foundation, Tokyo, 1963)

Natural Immunity, Noboro Muramoto (Oshawa Macrobiotic Foundation, Oroville, Ca., 1988)

Reversing Heart Disease, Julian Whitaker, MD (Warner Books, 1985)

Holistic Health, Lawrence Le Shan, MD (Holt Renechart, NY/Turnstone Press, UK, 1984)

Vital Facts About Foods, Otto Carque (Keats Publishing, New Canaan, Conn., 1975)

The Health Revolution (fourth ed.)**, Ross Horne (Happy Landings Publishers, Sydney, 1984)

*Improving On Pritikin**, Ross Horne (Happy Landings Publishers, Sydney, 1988)

The Anti-Cancer, Anti-Heart Attack Cookbook, Toni Bobbin, Ross Horne

Cancer

A Cancer Therapy, Results of Fifty Cases*, Max Gerson, MD (The Gerson Institute, Bonita, California)

The Prime Cause and Prevention of Cancer*, Otto Warburg, MD Ph.D (The Cancer Control Society, Los Angeles, 1967)

The Survival Factor in Neoplastic & Viral Diseases*, William F. Koch, Ph.D MD (The Vanderkloot Press, Detroit, 1961)

A Solution To The Cancer Problem*, Cornelius Moerman, MD (Cornelius Moerman, Vlaardingen, Netherlands, 1962)

Cancer and Cure: A Doctor's Story, Eva Hill, MD (Bachman & Turner, London, 1976)

Nutrition & Cancer, Myron Winick, MD (John Viley & Sons Inc., 1977)

Fresh Hope With New Cancer Treatments, Maurice Finkel, B.Sc MS (Prentice Hall, New Jersey, 1984)

Winning The Fight Against Breast Cancer, Carlton Fredericks, Ph.D (Grosset & Dunlop, New York, 1977)

One Answer to Cancer, William Kelley, BA DDS MS (The Kelley Foundation, 1974)

The Cancer Scourge & How to Destroy It; The Treatment of Cancer Without Operation (1903); and *Reminiscences of An Old Physician* (1924), Robert Bell, MD (Health Seekers International, Pinetown, South Africa)

Cholesterol: Causing Cancer and More, Arthur Isbit, Ph.D (Health Publishing Co, Chula Vista, Ca., 1984)

How I Overcame Inoperable Cancer, Dr Wong Hon Sun (Exposition Press, 1975)

How I Healed My Cancer Holistically, Dore Deverell (Psychenutrition Inc, Manhattan Beach, Ca., 1978)

Recalled By Life*, Anthony Satillaro, MD (Houghton Mifflin, Boston, 1982)

Cancer: A Healing Crisis, Jack Tropp (Exposition Press, NY, 1980)

You Bet You Can, Moscato Cards, (1984)

The Psychogenic Biochemical Aspects of Cancer, Harold Simmons (Physogenic Publishing Co., Sacramento, California, 1979)

Metabolic Ecology, A Way to Win the Cancer War, Fred Rohe (Wedgestone Press, 1982)

Prevention & Cure of Cancer, Mulhim Hassan, MD (Exposition Press, NY, 1983)

Coping With Cancer, Dr Morton Walker (Devin Adair Publishers, Connecticut, 1985)

Cancer & Vitamin C, Ewan Cameron & Linus Pauling (Warner Books, 1979)

The Cancer Blackout, Nat Morris (Regent House, 1977)

The Grape Cure, Basil Shackleton (Thorsons Publishing, 1969)

What You Can Do to Prevent Cancer, Dr Oliver Alabaster (Nelson Publishing, Australia, 1985, Simon & Schuster, NY)

The Treatment of Cancer With Herbs, John Heinerman (Biworld Publishers, Utah, 1980)

Cancer As A Turning Point, Lawrence Le Shan, Ph.D (Dutton, NY, 1989)

I Fought Leukemia and Won, Rex B. Eyre (Hawkes Publishing, Salt Lake City, 1982)

Is Cancer Curable? (Health Research, Mokelumne Hill, California)

Cancer Prevention Made Easy, Robert Schneider, MD (Prentice Hall, 1984)

You Can Conquer Cancer, Dr Ian Gawler (Hill of Content, Melbourne, 1984)

Getting Well Again, Carl Simonton, MD (J.P. Tarcher Inc., 1978)

I Beat Cancer, Bernice Wallin (Contemporary Books, 1978)

Vision Victory via Vitamins, Vital Foods, Diana Deimel (Chairu Publications, Pasadena, 1980)

Victory Over Cancer, Leonie McNabb (Veritas Publishing, 1978)

The Greatest Battle, Ronald Glasser, MD (Collins, London, 1978)

You Can Fight For Your Life, Lawrence LeShan MD PhD (Evans & Co., New York, 1977)

Cancer Winner: How I Purged Myself of Melanoma, Jacki Davison (Pacific Press, Peirce City, Mo., 1977)

The Anti Cancer Diet, Donald Germann, MD (Wyden Books, 1977)

Cancer: How To Prevent It, George Berkely, Ph.D (Prentice Hall, 1978)

How I Conquered Cancer Naturally, Eydie Mae (Harvest House Publishers, 1975)

Healed of Cancer, Jo Lawson (Logos International, 1977)

Cancer Causes & Natural Controls, Lynn Dallin, Ph.D (Ashley Books, Port Washington, 1983)

Cancer: A Disease of Civilization, Vilhjalmur Stephansson (Hill & Wang, New York, 1960)

Cancer and Other Diseases from Meat Consumption, Blanche Leonardo, Ph.D (Leaves of Healing Publications, Santa Monica, 1979)

An End To Cancer?, Dr Leon Chaitow (Thorsons Publishers, 1983)

Does Diet Cure Cancer?, Dr Maud Tresillian Fore, MD (Thorsons Publishers, 1971)

The Grape Cure, Johanna Brandt (Ehret Literature Publishing Co., Beaumont, Ca., 1948)

Be Your Own Doctor, Dr Ann Wigmore (Hemisphere Press, NY, 1976)

Cancer: A Disease of Civilization, Ebba Waerland (The Provoker Press, St Catherine, Ontario, 1976)

Too Young to Die, Rick Hill (Hill Publications, Grand Rapids, 1979)

Victory Over Cancer Without Radium or Surgery, Cyril Scott (Health Science Press, UK, 1939, 3rd impression 1969)

You Don't Have To Die*, Dr Harry S. Hoxsey (Nature Heals, Chapala, Mexico, 1956)

Healing Miracles From Macrobiotics, Jean Charles Kohler (Parker Publishing, W. Nyack, NY, 1979)

The Cancer Syndrome, Ralph Moss (Grove Press, NY, 1980)

Anatomy of An Illness, Norman Cousins (Norton, 1979; Bantam, 1981)

The Power of Positive Thinking, Norman Vincent Peale (Prentice Hall, 1952)

Mind-Made Disease, Ahri Vijayedev Yogendra (Yoga Education Centre, St Kilda, Melbourne, 1977)

AIDS

Note: Readers on AIDS should include as desirable reading all the books, particularly those on cancer.

AIDS The HIV Myth*, Jad Adams (Macmillan, 1989)

Roger's Recovery from AIDS*, Bob Owen, MD (DAVAR, Ca., 1987)

They Conquered AIDS, Scott J. Gregory, Bianca Leonardo (Free Of Life Publications, Ca., 1989)

Healing AIDS Naturally*, Laurence Badgley, MD (Human Energy Press, San Bruno, 1987)

Beyond AIDS: A Journey Into Healing, George Nelton (Brotherhood Press, Ca., 1988)

Conquering AIDS NOW! With Natural Treatment, Scott J. Gregory, Bianca Leonardo (Warner Books, 1986)

You Can Knock Out AIDS, Ian Brighthope, MD (Biocentres, Melbourne, Australia, 1987)

AIDS & Syphilis: The Hidden Link, Harris Coulter, Ph.D (N. Atlantic Books, Berkeley, Ca., 1987)

AIDS & Substance Abuse, Larry Siegel, MD (Harrington Park Press, 1987)

Choose To Live*, Laurence Badgley, MD (Human Energy Press, 1987)

The AIDS Book: Creating A Positive Approach, Louise Hay (Hay House Inc., Santa Monica, 1988)

Death Rush, Poppers and AIDS, John Lauritsen, Hank Wilson (Pagan Press, NY, 1986)

AIDS: Hope Hoax and Hoopla*, Michael Culbert, D.Sc (The Robert Bradford Foundation, Chula Vista, Ca., 1989)

The Great AIDS Hoax, T.C. Fry (Life Science Institute, Austin, 1989)

AIDS Inc. Scandal of the Century, John Rappoport (Human Energy Press, San Bruno, 1988)

AIDS: A Comprehensive Investigation*, Margot Fromer (Pinnacle Books, NY, 1983)

Why I Survived AIDS, Niro Markoff Assistant with Paul Kelly (Simon & Schuster, 1991)

Psychoimmunity & The Healing Process, Jason Serinus (ed.) (Celestial Arts, Berkeley, Ca., 1986)

Index

Other Books by Ross Horne

LONGEVITY is easy...
Banish the diseases of civilisation,
HEART ATTACK, CANCER, ARTHRITIS and the rest are
Simple to explain, Simple to eliminate...
Follow **NATHAN PRITIKIN...JOIN**

THE
HEALTH
REVOLUTION
FOURTH EDITION

Revised and Enlarged Edition
Exciting NEW information on ...
Nutrition
Food Enzymes
Rejuvenation
Cancer
AIDS
Cot Deaths

Ross Horne

IMPROVING
ON
PRITIKIN—
YOU CAN DO BETTER!

— Ross Horne
author of THE HEALTH REVOLUTION

Read how Grain foods (cereals) burden the digestion, cause acidosis
and impure blood, the chief factors in skin disorders,
arthritis, cancer and other metabolic problems.

THE HEALTH REVOLUTION

Over 100,000 copies sold

ROSS HORNE · TONI BOBBIN
Anti-Cancer
Anti-Heart Attack
COOKBOOK
Feel great and live longer

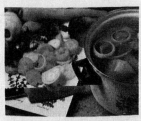

PRITIKIN DIET · GERSON DIET
LOW CHOLESTEROL DIET